The Widower's Journey

The Widower's Journey

HELPING MEN REBUILD AFTER THEIR LOSS

Herb Knoll

with Deborah Carr, Ph.D. & Robert L. Frick

A book for widowers and those who care about them

Dedication

To Michelle, who taught everyone how to care more about others.

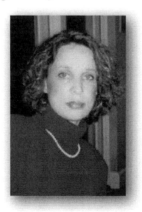

To Maria, who healed my heart and showed me how to love again, and whose support made the writing of this book possible.

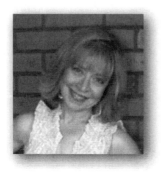

Contents

Acknowledgments

To this book's contributing widowers, who demonstrated tremendous courage by sharing their stories so that others may benefit. *The Widower's Journey* is our book.

To Deborah Carr, Ph.D., whose guidance was as valuable as the expert content she provided. To book editor Robert L. Frick, who helped organize and manage this project over a nine-year period. And to Walter G. Meyer for his review of this book's manuscript.

To the team of subject matter experts whose services better enabled *The Widower's Journey* to achieve its mission of providing comfort and support to widowers for years to come, especially Diedre Wachbrit-Braverman, Esq.; Mark Colgan, CFP; Justin T. Denney, Ph.D.; Rev. Gregg Elliott; Pastor Doug Fultz; Sofia Guzman, Esq.; Jennifer Ferguson, CFP; Pastor Kenny Hagin; Rabbi Alexis Pearce; Joseph Walsh, CFP; and Edward F. Zimmer, M.A.

To my children who supported me throughout the nine years of research and writing, I give my heartfelt appreciation. To my two beautiful daughters, Jessica R. Birkholz and Lauren C. Munyard, and my two bonus children, Michelle's son Jacques M. Everly and Maria's daughter Ingrid Delgado. I love you all.

About the Widowers Support Network

The *Widowers Support Network* was founded by author Herb Knoll in 2014 to comfort and assist widowers across America and around the world.

Participate: Your thoughts, suggestions, and opinions are welcome. Widowers and non-widowers alike are encouraged to register on our website and participate in the network's blog. See www.WidowersSupportNetwork.com.

You can also follow us on Facebook at *Widowers Support Network* and on Twitter: *@WidowersJourney*.

Purchase Books: To order multiple copies or bulk quantities of *The Widower's Journey*, contact the Widowers Support Network at 615.579.8136 or write *herb@WidowersSupportNetwork.com*

Custom-branded covers and private-label forewords written by representatives of sponsoring organizations and firms are available.

About the Widowers Support Network

The Widowers Support Network was founded by author Herb Knoll in 2014 to comfort and assist widowers across America and around the world.

Participate: Your thoughts, suggestions, and opinions are welcome. Widowers and non-widowers alike are encouraged to register on our website and participate in the network's blog. See www.WidowersSupportNetwork.com.

In addition to our website, the Widowers Support Network offers additional resources which can be very helpful to a grieving widower and those who love them including:

Widowers Support Network – Members Only: (Found on Facebook) A favorite yet confidential and exclusive group page available to widowed men, male caregivers who are caring for a seriously ill or terminally ill spouse and subject matter experts (sorry ladies, males only) who donate their services to the group's membership. (A free service)

Widowers Support Network: (Found on Facebook) Open to the general public, the *Widowers Support Network* on Facebook provides information, news you can use and helpful tips on how to overcome the challenges of becoming a widower. This is an ideal resource for family members and friends of widowed men. (A free service)
You can also follow us on Twitter: *@WidowersJourney*.

Purchase Books: To order multiple copies or bulk quantities of *The Widower's Journey*, contact the Widowers Support Network at 615.579.8136 or write *herb@WidowersSupportNetwork.com*
Custom-branded covers and private-label forewords written by representatives of sponsoring organizations and firms are available.

Herb Knoll the Speaker: To schedule Herb Knoll to speak at your next meeting, conference, or convention, contact him at 615.579.8136 or write him at *herb@WidowersSupportNetwork.com*.

Introduction

"She's gone," the nurse said. I tried to grasp that my wife of sixteen years, Michelle, had died. Until that moment Michelle had been a presence, and now she was forever absent. Then my first few moments of bereavement were cut short. "Mr. Knoll," the nurse said, "What are you going to do with her remains?"

Michelle had fought cancer for thirty-nine months, but not once had I considered what would happen after she passed. Her moments alive were gifts, and the time she was with me was so precious that even when her body was wasting away, I did not squander one moment thinking about her final resting place. And besides, I hadn't lived in San Antonio long enough to figure out my preferred barber, let alone how I would care for Michelle's "remains."

"I don't know," I told her.

The nurse craned her neck to look at the clock on the wall above the nurse's station. "Your insurance won't cover her after midnight, so you need to have her moved within three hours."

I was alone, grief-stricken, exhausted, and in a new city. My wife lay dead before me. I had 180 minutes—make that 176 minutes—to fulfill my first duty as a widower. So I went to the *Yellow Pages* to find someone—anyone—who could come and take both Michelle and me away from that bitter place.

And so began my widower's journey. Those first few minutes after Michelle's death foreshadowed what lay ahead: dealing with loss, taking practical steps, and seeking others who could help me. Also overcoming barriers. This book was written to help other widowers on their own journey to recovery and serve as a roadmap to help navigate all those issues with practical advice from experts and fellow widowers.

Although this isn't a book about me, I will share steps in my journey at times to help guide you through your own experiences. My hope is that you will learn from my successes and my mistakes, and that you'll know you're not alone in what you're feeling and what you're dealing with. Yes, we'll talk at times about feelings—a tough subject for many men—but the emphasis will be on equipping you for a successful journey to recovery.

I managed the journey, found happiness again, and eventually remarried. I've interviewed dozens of widowers who successfully navigated their own journeys; you will meet them in this book. I've also interviewed experts with special knowledge that can help widowers. We will travel together with you as guides along your path to happiness.

Why Widowers?

If you have this book in your hands, you are likely among the 2.7 million widowers in the United States, and perhaps one of the 420,000 men who became widowers this year. That means there is also a good chance that, like me, you could find no resources to help you navigate your own journey to rebuilding your life. This book addresses the challenges of men who have lost their spouses. And we men need the help. Consider these facts:

- Widowers have a higher suicide risk. According to studies, they arc anywhere from almost twice as likely (*Social Science Quarterly*, December 2009) to three times as likely (*Social Science Medicine*, 1995) as married men to commit suicide. The risk is even higher for widowers who are either younger or older. Those over age 75 are ten times more likely than widows to commit suicide, and widowers under 35 are seventeen times more likely to commit suicide than married men (*American Journal of Public Health*, 2002).

- Widowers are more likely than married men to die in an accident or from alcohol-related causes, lung cancer, or heart disease during the first six months following their loss.

- When men are widowed, they often slip into bad behaviors, such as driving recklessly, drinking, smoking, and eating unhealthily. These behaviors, combined with the tremendous stress from loss, take a toll on men's health and life spans.

- Dozens of academic studies show that widowers have poorer mental and physical health than their married counterparts.

- Widowers are often vulnerable to scam artists and predators, including unscrupulous wannabe mates, financial advisors, and even family members and caretakers. In *The Widower's Journey*, you'll meet a widower who had $1.4 million hijacked by a predator who pretended to fall in love with him.

- Widowers contribute to the high cost of healthcare and add to taxpayers' burdens because of high rates of poor health and succumbing to new or re-emerging addictions.

At first, I was surprised by these statistics, but then it occurred to me that I had experienced and witnessed the root causes of these problems firsthand. To write this book I interviewed many fellow widowers, and I found that these men were often reluctant to discuss their grief or to seek help. And that behavior lies at the heart of many of the problems listed above. It can be traced back to our childhoods, when we were told that "boys don't cry" and we should "just suck it up." We'll talk about this programming and how we can fight it together so that we can help widowers in future generations. I've seen the power of men working together to help their fellow widowers, and once we identify these challenges, I'm convinced we can overcome them.

In a few cases, widowers who had agreed to be interviewed later withdrew their cooperation. One told me that even speaking about the circumstances surrounding the passing of his wife was too painful. He didn't want to be reminded of the events that led up to her death, some of the darkest days of his life. Another said he thought that revealing his story would be a sign of weakness—an Achilles heel for many men. A third widower had moved on to a new relationship and didn't want to risk harming it by allowing me to write about his marriage. That's symptomatic of another challenge that widowers face: managing new relationships while honoring the memories of their late wives. We will address these attitudes, as well as damaging stereotypes held by friends, family, and even new romantic partners—stereotypes such as men rebound more quickly because they're less emotional.

The statistics paint a grim picture, but the majority of widowers will bounce back. Academic studies and many of the men I spoke with show that most rediscover happiness—sometimes with a new partner, sometimes alone. As sociologist and internationally recognized bereavement expert Deborah Carr has written, widowers (and widows) are resilient. They find happiness and personal growth, and they even discover new facets of themselves after the initial grief fades. But as the statistics attest, that doesn't mean the road is smooth or free from collateral damage. My goal is to help make that road easier and reduce the harm suffered by widowers and by those around them.

When it comes to unearthing the ways in which the loss of a life partner affects men in all aspects of their lives, *The Widower's Journey* leaves no stone unturned. To bring you the best research on grief and recovery, I've partnered with Dr. Carr and recruited a team of experts on a wide range of relevant topics, both academics, and practitioners. In addition, the dozens of widowers from across the country I have interviewed have shared trials and triumphs that readers will readily identify with and learn from.

The Widower's Journey delves into the lives of men who found a way not just to survive, but to thrive. What distinguishes these widowers from those who don't find healing? Often, those who struggle simply don't have the right information. So this book provides detailed advice from experts on grief, loneliness, physical and mental health, employment, parenting, relationships, and much more.

Beyond helping individual widowers, which is the main goal of this book, I have a grander goal. By underscoring the unique needs of widowers generally, *The Widower's Journey* will help create supportive communities for grieving men and those who love them. Part of that is addressing the larger issues of how society often fails widowers and how society can change to help them. I'll work to create those communities and address these larger problems, and I will continue to speak to widower groups. To learn more, be sure to register with the Widowers Support Network on its website (www.WidowersSupportNetwork.com) and follow the network on Facebook and Twitter (@WidowersJourney).

Ancient Chinese philosopher Lao Tzu famously said, "A journey of 1,000 miles begins with a single step." And I'd like to share the first steps of my journey with you now. As I said, this book isn't about me, but I hope knowing where I've been will encourage you to let me help you with your journey.

Michelle's Last Days

The battle for Michelle's life began on Christmas Eve 2004, when she was diagnosed with pancreatic cancer. It ended on a rainy Friday night at San Antonio's Methodist Hospital just after 9 p.m., on March 7, 2008. The death watch had begun two days earlier, when Michelle's oncologist told her, "We have a plan." During the previous three weeks, she had developed a condition known as pleural effusion, which causes impaired breathing. Three surgeries couldn't fix it. The "plan" meant removing the tube that had been draining fluids from her chest. Then, in a day or two, Michelle's lungs wouldn't be able to expand, and death would come.

Michelle told the doctor she feared feeling as though she was suffocating. To allay her fears and provide her as much comfort as possible, he prescribed doses of liquid morphine. Administering it became my responsibility. I dreaded it, but I knew it would provide Michelle some peace during her final hours.

I would place the tip of a syringe in the corner of Michelle's mouth to deliver the morphine. At times, Michelle would grit her teeth to prevent me from doing what no one should ever have to do for someone they love. She was heavily sedated and unable to speak, but I could imagine what she was thinking: "Why are you doing this to me? You're killing me." The doctors told me that Michelle was so sedated she wouldn't realize what was happening. But the expression I saw on her face after I gave her each dose haunts me still, as does the guilt from doing it.

A few family members and close friends stayed with me at Michelle's bedside beginning on Thursday morning and remained with me until Michelle passed on Friday. She was 52.

After she died—and the nurse had served the eviction notice—the others left so that I could spend a few minutes alone with Michelle in the dimly lit hospital room. Then it hit me that my beautiful bride was gone. The joys we shared were now only memories. I wasn't crying because I had exhausted my supply of tears. I noticed the sign I had posted on the wall that read, "Jesus will never leave you, nor will I."

I took a moment to hug Michelle, and I discovered that she had developed bedsores across her back. She never complained about them, which was typical of her. I knew that bedridden patients were at risk of developing bedsores, and I simultaneously became angry that the nursing staff allowed the sores to form and guilty that I had failed to examine her myself.

Within minutes of Michelle's passing, I felt as though I had let her down by not properly caring for her. But I buried those feelings to manage the task at hand.

What an Angel Left Behind

Yes, "She's gone." But she will never be forgotten by the many lives she touched.

Michelle was a beautiful woman of Ukrainian heritage who was at ease anywhere. Her blue-green eyes, chestnut hair, and flawless complexion turned heads. I was a banker, and Michelle often accompanied me to business events. Some were black-tie, some were casual get-togethers with clients, but Michelle navigated every room with ease, engaging strangers in conversation by just offering one of her trademark smiles.

If something interested Michelle, she dived in headfirst. When she didn't like some of the decisions our local government was making when we lived in East Greenbush, N.Y., she ran for office on the Republican ticket. When she fell short by just 27 votes, she asked me to take her to the Democratic election headquarters so that she could congratulate her opponent. As Michelle entered the hall, all of her opponent's supporters broke into applause for Michelle, a woman they had come to learn was truly extraordinary.

One day, at my office in San Antonio, a female staff member told me how Michelle's courage inspired her to renew the chemotherapy treatments she had discontinued. She said, "Michelle has given me a reason to live and hope for a cure." She wanted me to express her gratitude to Michelle, who was hospitalized and near death at the time.

Michelle was a bright light, whether serving as vice president of the New York State Dental Assistants Association, volunteering at a senior citizen center, leading a group of Cub Scouts, serving as a team mom for her son's baseball team, entertaining bank clients with me, or being the guest of Matilda Cuomo, wife of Governor Mario Cuomo, in the Governor's box at the Saratoga Race Track.

Michelle adored her only child, Jacques, as well as the three pedigreed golden retrievers she bred—Caroline, Spencer, and Charlotte. I used to tease Michelle, saying, "Every time a golden puppy is born, I go further down the list of important people—or dogs—in your life."

Michelle was skilled at crafts, from quilting blankets to making fine needle points. She spent hundreds of hours making large China dolls, crafting them in the exact image of the recipient; she made one for my granddaughter Alyssa Birkholz. She was always working on a gift for someone, and among our immediate family and friends her works remain on display as cherished keepsakes.

My sister, Sandy Cowan, once said, "You'd have to be careful around Michelle when shopping. If you mentioned that you liked something you saw in a store, it would later appear at the front door of your home or under your pillow without so much as a note attached."

Between 2002 and 2007, we lived in Brentwood, Tennessee, a suburb of Nashville. It was during this period that once a week,

Michelle and her best friend Joanne Smith volunteered at a senior center located in nearby Franklin, Tennessee. There they led a craft class for older women (also known as The Ladies of Franklin) who lived in subsidized housing nearby. But her attention to those women didn't stop there. Each week, Michelle would bring food for the ladies to take home and feed to their families. The Ladies of Franklin came to Michelle's memorial service to pay their last respects, all sitting in the front pew.

On Valentine's Day 2008, Michelle was scheduled to have fluid drained from her chest. When I entered the kitchen for my first cup of coffee, I found her busy on her latest project: making pretzel sticks dipped in various flavors of chocolate, each stick beautifully wrapped in heart-themed cellophane, with a red or pink bow. "These are Valentine's Day gifts for your staff," she said. "Employees always like getting gifts from their boss." We didn't know at that moment that this would be the last thing she did at home before entering the hospital for the last time. How fitting that it was an act to please others.

Michelle's crowning acts of generosity happened each time she visited Vanderbilt-Ingram Cancer Center in Nashville, where she received treatments. As we would sit in the waiting room, Michelle would often ask, "Who is helping that patient over there?" She'd say how fortunate we were to have friends, family, and good health insurance. "But what about them? Who do they have? We have to find a way to help them." It was her concern for others that inspired me to start the Michelle's Angels Foundation, a not-for-profit organization with the mission to "Provide Love, Hope, Compassion and Comforting Music to Those Who Quietly Suffer." The Michelle's Angels Foundation is Michelle's spirit in charity form. Supported by a team of volunteers and singer-songwriters, the Michelle's Angels Foundation performs various acts of charity and concerts at homes for battered women, cancer treatment centers, cardiac care units, pediatric wards, hospice centers, and similar venues. To learn more, visit www.MichellesAngels.com or Michelle's Angels Foundation, Inc. on Facebook.

My Promise

After finding a funeral home to accept Michelle, I walked to my car in the Methodist Hospital parking garage. It was the loneliest walk of my life, and when I arrived home, I realized it was no longer *our* home, it was just a house filled with memories. And it was once filled with Michelle's laughter, never to be heard again. It still held her fragrance, now never to be enjoyed. I was about to begin the next phase of my life, but I was paralyzed by uncertainty and saw no path into the future.

I was a banker; I didn't know how to be a widower. But I knew the power of good advice and had relied on it from mentors and books throughout my career. Within a few weeks of Michelle's memorial service, I went to my local Barnes and Noble to buy a book about how to put my life back on track after becoming a widower. I didn't find anything on the shelves, so I asked a clerk, who entered "widower" into his computer to see what was available. He looked up from the screen and said, "Mister, I don't have a damn thing for you." I went home and Googled the topic for myself. I found a few books, each of which was an accounting of one man's experience. The only other book was an academic work published in 1996, not a practical guide.

I didn't need theory. I needed direction that could help me overcome my challenges. It was that day I made a promise to myself that once I had found my way through those challenges, I would write a guide for widowers so they wouldn't feel as helpless as I did. I was inspired by Michelle's example of always helping others in need, and I felt she would want me to use my experiences to help my fellow man, just as she had used her experiences fighting cancer to help others facing the same battle.

I knew first that I had to heal myself. But during my own journey I carefully noted all the challenges I faced, and later I interviewed dozens of other widowers to record their challenges. Like all widowers, I found myself enrolled in the accelerated graduate degree program for widowed men. There is no campus, nor a classroom, but I promised myself I would write this guidebook.

CHAPTER 1

Caring for Your Terminally Ill Wife

know this book will be bought mainly by, and for, men following the deaths of their wives. But the pain of loss often strikes before death. *Anticipatory grief* refers to the feelings of loss that we feel when we gradually see a loved one slipping away. For this reason, my hope is that the advice in this chapter will reach men who are caring for terminally ill spouses. I learned many lessons the hard way during my time as a caregiver, as did other widowers I've spoken with, and I'd be remiss if I didn't share these lessons. If you are reading this after your wife's death, you may want to skip now to Chapter 2, which begins our path on dealing with grief, though you may find some solace in reading this chapter about what others have experienced as caregivers.

Men who do the right things when helping terminally ill spouses not only are better caregivers but can also heal more quickly after their wife is lost. Furthermore, those who take the right financial and legal actions before the death of their wife will start their recovery with more money in the bank and an estate in better order. Those who are prepared to carry out their wife's preferences for end-of-life medical treatments are less likely to have painful disagreements with family members, who may want to impose their own values on that care. So this chapter will give advice about everything from helping your children to getting medical care to making the right financial and legal moves.

The Best Medical Care

Let's start with the most immediate, critical issue: No one should settle for less than the best medical care. Many widowers I've interviewed live with regret because they feel they had not been aggressive enough in seeking top care. So take charge of your mate's care. Don't be like so many who do whatever the doctor tells them—I've found this to be particularly true among older widowers, who I think have been more conditioned to accept what the medical establishment tells them. Search for the best care, and challenge recommendations. Fight the good fight for your spouse.

One of the first things Michelle said after receiving her diagnosis: "Find me the best surgeon you can." I didn't want the second best for her, either, so I turned to my business skills to research best practices and find the best doctors to treat her condition. I discovered that Michelle was eligible to have a risky but possibly lifesaving surgery known as the Whipple Procedure. This is a radical, ten-hour operation involving removing parts of several organs. It requires a surgeon with great skill, and in our search for such a doctor, Michelle and I first met with the only surgeon at the Vanderbilt-Ingram Cancer Center at that time who could perform it. He said he'd done it 65 times over the previous three years.

Next, I contacted the University of Texas MD Anderson Cancer Center in Houston. It is regularly ranked as the top hospital for cancer care in the United States (most recently, in 2016, by *U.S. News & World Report*). It had six surgeons who performed three Whipple procedures *per week*. That sealed it. We were going to MD Anderson.

As we were submitting our admission papers, I learned that the top surgeon was Dr. Doug Evans. But the intake rep said, "You won't find him assigned to your wife's case. He's booked solid. In fact, you'll be lucky if you get surgeon number six."

So I began asking everyone I knew if they had any influence at MD Anderson. As it turned out, I had three connections. I got them to all work on our behalf. Soon I got a call from MD Anderson, saying, "Dr. Evans wants to see Michelle tomorrow in Houston." *Hallelujah.*

I understand I was lucky to have health insurance and the contacts which helped Michelle get admitted to MD Anderson. But what does a devoted husband do if he wants to secure the best possible care for his ailing wife and he doesn't enjoy the contacts others have? I presented this question to Jennifer Kennedy-Stovall, Director of Patient Access Support Services at MD Anderson.

"Every patient needs an advocate—one that will never worry if they are being too pushy or intrusive," said Kennedy-Stovall. "We continually hear from patients and advocates who feel a need to apologize to us for being too difficult, especially with those who might soon be providing the needed medical care. All patients or advocates should feel free to do what they must, even at the risk of having to call our offices four times each day regarding what others may view as trivial matters."

Kennedy-Stovall encourages husbands to ask around for assistance if they are unable to serve as their wife's advocate. Ask your family, friends, colleagues, or fellow parishioners at your house of worship if they can help secure the desired care. When a loved one is seriously ill, no obstacle should make you surrender.

"And should the patient learn her case is not accepted, be sure to ask, 'Then who can I talk to here that can assist me in securing care elsewhere?' " said Kennedy-Stovall. "Many if not most hospitals have staff whose purpose it is to assist those seeking care to find it elsewhere—and quickly."

Widower John Heffernan had the right attitude when he served as Mary's advocate: "My style is to take charge. I don't trust health-care systems to best manage anyone's care, so I intended to manage Mary's care myself. She had metastasis cancer, and the prognosis for that is never good. I felt we might have a year to enjoy. We lived each of next five years she had like it was the last year."

Widower Jeff Gower put it succinctly: "This was our cancer, not just Susan's, so that's the way we treated it."

But many widowers, like Harold Moran, have regrets. "I wanted to find a hospital or program that specialized in cancer treatment, but I didn't. I question if I gave my wife Connie every chance I could to beat her disease. I still second-guess myself."

Being a good advocate is about more than seeking the best care. As I said, not everyone has the means to pay for care at a top-notch hospital. Others lack the ties to prominent physicians. But many aspects of being a good advocate don't cost a dime.

Several of our contributing widowers spoke strongly about keeping great records. I couldn't agree more. Widower John Von Der Haar found his binder indispensable. "I always had it with me and was surprised at the number of times I used it, either for information about a prescription, prior appointment, last date of Mary's MRI, etc. I took responsibility for something she should not have to worry about."

So buy a loose-leaf binder with tabs and plastic sheets to hold business cards. Buy Post-It notes, markers, highlighters, and lined paper. Keep track of each contact and take detailed notes. Establish a separate tab for each hospital, clinic, radiology, pharmacy, social worker, etc. The computer-savvy can create spreadsheets and other documents so that all the information is easy to search. Always secure a copy of the doctor's notes following a visit, and be sure to ask for digital copies of all scans, x-rays, MRIs, and other tests.

And don't assume your wife is taking her medicine properly. Some wives are so medicated they don't know whether they took their drugs at the proper time or in the proper dose. Older wives who may be showing early signs of dementia or cognitive impairment might not remember taking their medication earlier in the day, and they may accidentally take double the dose.

Binder Items

- A list of your wife's prescriptions, including the dosages, the schedule for taking them, and the illness for which each was prescribed. Keep a list of medical reactions to watch out for.
- A directory of all medical contacts, including physicians, nurses, nurse's aides, technicians, social workers, and anyone else you might need to contact.
- A list of people, including friends and family, whom you will need to keep informed about your spouse's condition. An excellent way to do so is to establish a page at www. CaringBridge.org, which can be a source of information for those people.
- Monthly calendars with enough room for appointments and notes.
- A section to record payments and the mileage driven for appointments. (Remember, medical expenses may be tax-deductible.)
- Copies of your wife's various ID cards (health insurance, pharmacy, dental plan, and employment).
- Copies of pertinent sections of your health insurance policies, definitions, descriptions, and co-payments.
- Sections for medical questions and billing questions.

You might want to make duplicates and give copies of these files to a trusted friend, neighbor, or adult child. These backup files can be essential if you are traveling or become ill or infirmed yourself.

I'll add a personal note here about the care that goes beyond medical care. Carefully monitor your wife's exposure to media. One evening, Michelle and I decided to take in a movie. Once in line, I realized I had made a terrible mistake and had bought tickets for the popular movie titled *The Bucket List*. In this film, two men suffering from cancer travel around the world to live out their "bucket lists" of adventures before they die. Clearly, a bad choice. I found the theater manager, who let me exchange my tickets for another film. At home, I found I would often change the television channel if the program or news broadcast involved cancer, death, or sad storylines.

When your wife has a dire illness, don't be a victim. Be a fighter. Yes, it is a fight you may lose, but the act of fighting has many benefits and is a victory in itself. For example, anxiety comes from feelings of dread and helplessness, among other things, and you can diminish anxiety by taking charge. As long as you are contributing to the care of your wife and can remain hopeful for a good outcome, you're also taking care of your own mental well-being.

Embrace your bias for action—it's something I think men particularly benefit from doing. Men are wired to be fixers. For example, when my brother Don and his wife, Kathy, were on a plane, a young boy seated behind Kathy kept kicking the back of her seat. Kathy leaned over and mentioned it to Don. Immediately, Don looked back and told the young man, "Knock it off." Kathy was chagrined.

"Why did you do that?" she said. "I didn't ask you to say anything; I just wanted to tell you what was happening." Even so, fixing things gives use a sense of purpose, and it relieves a lot of frustration.

But being a good fighter also means knowing when to stop the fight, according to Rutgers University sociology professor Deborah Carr. If medical treatments are no longer helping, or if your loved one is tired of fighting and suffering and is ready to go, it may be time to accept the reality of her impending death and enjoy moments of love, peace, calm, and acceptance. Hospice care is one of the best services available for dying patients, as it focuses on providing them with comfort after the decision is made to stop aggressive treatments.

In our own case, knowing we had done everything we could to get her the best care, Michelle and I decided we should live our lives and trust God to take care of the rest. "Let's try to have normal lives," Michelle would say.

Speaking of God, don't discount the importance that faith can have on your wife's positive outlook, which is a critical ingredient in fighting illness. If you are a believer in the existence of a higher power, be sure to involve your church, synagogue, or other house of worship in your wife's care. As Michelle use to say, "God will have his way." So firm was Michelle's faith that she consistently took comfort in knowing her Lord was at her side. There is no doubt Michelle's faith helped her live as normal a life as possible during the months she fought cancer. And I know my faith was crucial to helping my mental health when caring for Michelle. (Chapter 5 is devoted to matters of faith.)

Even if you are a non-believer, or don't actively practice your faith, you can help your wife tend to her faith by taking her to her house of worship, getting her religious leader to visit her, and observing religious rituals. Don't miss a beat, because regardless of whether your wife survives or she loses her battle, she will want to have her God's graces. Some ailing spouses are reluctant to involve their religious community because they feel it might make their husbands uncomfortable. If you think this describes your situation, put your feelings aside.

And beyond religious practice, there are other ways to help your wife keep the faith. Shortly after my wife's diagnosis, widower Brian Jakes called me. I took his call from my car so that Michelle would not overhear our conversation. Brian lost his wife, Lucy, when she was only 46. Brian knew all too well the challenges that lie ahead for me, and he wanted to offer some coaching. While Brian provided me with much sage advice, one piece stood out: "Always speak in future tense." He said doing that would show Michelle that I was committed to her recovery and making plans to share life with her for years to come.

And never forget about your wife's femininity. Following Michelle's surgery, I searched for a way to pamper her. I walked Houston's nearby business district until I found a salon that did manicures. While the manicurists typically didn't work outside of the shop, I convinced the salon to send one of them to the hospital so that she could give Michelle a manicure and pedicure. Michelle loved it.

Widower Harold Moran told us how his late wife Connie's daughters would comfort her by brushing her hair. "We took every chance we could to do that for her. I believe it helped her a great deal."

I knew that traveling back and forth to Vanderbilt-Ingram Cancer Center and occasional trips to MD Anderson in Houston were tough for Michelle because she was in pain. One day when I drove home from the hospital, I went over a small dip in the road slowly, but she cried out that it hurt her down to her bones. So I sold my car and leased another that had a smoother ride.

If your wife is receiving chemo or radiation, she may lose her hair. Be sure you pick up any hair from her pillow or that falls on the bathroom floor, tub or shower. Clean her brushes and combs of excessive amounts of hair when she is not around to observe your efforts.

Also, plan vacations or special events for both the near and the distant future. Some researchers have even found that having a special event to look forward to can extend dying patients' lives by days or weeks. My editor, Bob Frick, told me of a critically ill neighbor who managed to live to be with her daughter at her bat mitzvah, then died two days later. Emory sociologist Ellen Idler conducted a now-famous study that found terminally ill Christians would often survive until just past Christmas, and that dying Jewish adults were more likely to pass slightly after, rather than before, their holidays. The power of future goals cannot be overstated. Encourage your wife to maintain her career, hobbies, and social calendar. Surround yourselves with people who are upbeat and positive.

Widower Norris Jergensen saw the importance of striving for normalcy. "I tried to be with Darlene as much as possible and got her what she needed when she needed it. I would take her to see our kids when she felt up to it. I'd go grocery shopping and run errands. I took her clothes shopping even though she would rarely buy anything because she would look into the mirror and not like what she saw."

Widower Keith Merriam gave Suzy a free rein. "Even when Suzy wanted to go dog-sledding at the time her breast cancer had metastasized to her bones, I agreed. She had the time of her life!"

And make love. Gravely ill spouses still have feelings and desires. Lovemaking may not sound tempting during treatment. But to deny your ill spouse the warmth and intimacy of love-making may suggest to her how you no longer find her attractive, or that your love for her may be fading.

Finally, don't be afraid to break some rules and take what some might consider drastic measures. Widower Brian Jakes took his twelve-year-old son out of school for a year. According to Brian, while their daughter was coping reasonably well with his wife Lucy's illness, their son needed to be with his mother, and the mother needed to be with her son. Brian received considerable criticism for this, but in retrospect, he believes it was the right decision.

Become Secretary of the Interior

You will need to take command of all of your household chores. Don't look to your ill wife to carry this load, unless she wants to as part of maintaining her routine. So take care of her part of the cooking, cleaning the home, shopping for groceries, and more if she is challenged by those chores or doesn't want to perform them. If you have children, give them some of those responsibilities. Doing so would likely let them feel less helpless and provide them some level of satisfaction that they are contributing to their mother's care.

Most critically ill people have trouble navigating stairs. If a one-story home or apartment is not in the cards, at least move your wife's bedroom to the first floor. Some folks accomplish this by converting their dining room to a first-floor bedroom. If there is no bathroom on the first floor, consider getting a portable toilet from a medical supply store. Widower Steve Marquardt created a "comfort zone" on the couch for his wife, Merethe, the children, and the family's German shepherd. "I would get up early and make sure all of her medicines were ready. I had all of her food and juice ready when she woke up. Anything she needed or wanted."

Recruit a Team of Angels

Now, you may think you can do everything yourself while main-taining a career. Get over that notion fast. I don't care how talented and resourceful you think you are; you'll need a team of angels. A great blessing Michelle and I received was our wonderful friends and neighbors, whom we affectionately referred to as Michelle's Angels (a handle we would later use when naming a not-for-profit founda-tion after Michelle). If you don't have friends and family nearby, you may want to check with your religious community or nearby support groups for people in your situation.

During the early stages of Michelle's cancer, I worked for Bank of America in Nashville, Tennessee. During this time, the Michelle's Angels team made a huge difference in our lives. It all started in early January 2005, just days before Michelle would have her surgery in Houston when I mentioned to her how she had angels all around her. Michelle asked, "What do you mean?"

I explained, "Everything you needed to happen for you to live is taking place. You were diagnosed early, you secured a top surgeon to treat you, and you have neighbors rallying around to support you." Everything had fallen into place.

Michelle's Angels included our neighbors in Brentwood, Tennessee, who virtually took over our home. From stocking our refrigerator to doing laundry, they surrounded her with love and compassion. Michelle bred golden retrievers and had a litter born the day after she was diagnosed. She was unable to care for the nine puppies, but neighbors took over and cared for them until they were sold eight weeks later.

One of the Michelle's Angels, Joanne Smith, stayed by Michelle's side through more than 100 chemotherapy and radiation treatments, chatting away or watching movies together. Joanne's loving deeds provided me the relief I needed so that I could perform my duties at the bank. One of the most important things caregivers need is respite. Ask a friend to help care for your wife if you feel you need a few hours off. And don't feel guilty if you use those hours to go to the gym, or even take quiet time to read a book. Caring for ourselves occasionally sustains and energizes us to care for others.

Watch Your Health

The psychological strain of being a caregiver is taxing, so caregivers need to take care of themselves, too. Take breaks regularly, and see a doctor routinely. During my time as a caregiver, I not only saw a doctor for my physical health, I also saw a psychiatrist at Vanderbilt Medical Center. I knew I needed to be at the top of my game and to be thinking clearly if I was to care properly for Michelle.

But even though I took the proper steps, I couldn't mitigate all the stress. Ten days after Michelle passed away, I was diagnosed with kidney stones that required surgery. Within a few years, I was diagnosed with prostate cancer. Were these conditions related to my serving as a caregiver? I'll never know for sure, but statistics on illnesses following traumatic events suggest they were. I'll talk more about widower health concerns in Chapter 4, which is devoted to that topic. As Dr. Carr will explain, popular lore is that new widowers may "die of a broken heart," but the truth is that they neglect their own health while giving care to their wives, and often they don't know that they themselves are sick until it's too late.

Paula Spencer Scott, a Caring.com contributing editor, says that caregivers report higher levels of psychological stress compared with non-caregivers, according to a 2011 report by the UCLA Center for Health Policy Research. "Caregivers are more likely than the general public to have a chronic illness (82% versus 61%). And the longer a caregiver is in the role, the more likely he or she is to report a decline in health."

Dr. Carr explains: "Caregiving can be very stressful, and the emotional and physical responses to that stress vary based on how emotionally and physically intense and long-term the caregiving is." She adds that the stress of caregiving can be compounded by other major stressors, such as exorbitant medical bills, having a difficult job, or simultaneously caring for an aging parent.

In later chapters, you will find advice on how to use employee assistance programs and the Family and Medical Leave Act (FMLA) to help you cope with physical and mental health issues, give you time to spend with your wife, and manage the situation.

Financial Moves

We go into finances at length in Appendix I, but here are some steps that can be taken while your wife is still alive that are worthwhile.

First, if you are a homeowner, apply for a home equity line of credit (HELOC). The equity you have in your home is a valuable asset and can be a significant financial tool to help you and your family through some rocky times. It's easier to get a HELOC when you still have your wife's income. A HELOC lets you have access to a large amount of money (depending on the amount of equity you have built up in your home) that you can use in case of an emergency. In most cases, the homeowner pays only after he has taken a cash advance against the preapproved line of credit. If you hunt around, you should be able to find one with no or low costs and a low-interest rate. Bankrate.com is an excellent source of information about the availability of HELOCs.

The time to apply for a home equity line of credit is *before* you need it, and when your household income is at its highest. That's because when you need it, you may no longer qualify to get one approved—or you won't be able to get as high a credit line as you want. I recommend that all couples (even those without a family crisis to deal with) apply for a HELOC. It may well be the best financial move you can make to protect your family.

Another thing to get before you need it: A low-cost life insurance policy for your spouse through your employer, if available. If possible, get the maximum amount of coverage. And if the employer makes the offer with no physical required, don't hesitate.

When I worked for Bank of America in Tennessee, I bought a spousal life insurance policy through Bank of America for Michelle. After I changed jobs and moved to San Antonio, it occurred to me that I should see whether I could keep the policy by converting it to one owned by Michelle. I could—though we barely made the 60-day deadline for conversion after leaving my old employer. The beauty of this transaction is that because it was an existing policy, Michelle wasn't required to take a physical. Having the policy in place helped me provide for Jacques, Michelle's son from her previous marriage, who was then 23.

Speaking of life insurance, here's a controversial move you could make: Essentially, you can cash in an existing life insurance policy with a "viatical life insurance settlement." Such settlements have disadvantages, but Certified Financial Planner Mark Colgan, a one-time widower, says they can be useful. The settlements provide terminally ill or chronically ill patients an opportunity to sell their life insurance policy to a third party for an amount that is set higher than the policy's cash surrender value but less than its face value. In such transactions, the original policyholder receives much-needed cash, perhaps to pay medical bills or other expenses. The third party becomes the policy owner and is responsible for all future premiums. Upon the death of the original policy holder, the policy death benefit is paid to the third party. But the cost for such a deal can be substantial, so check with a financial advisor to see if it makes sense to consider.

Legal Considerations

When your wife has a serious illness, you'll be asked to make tough medical decisions on her behalf. Or perhaps she will want another party to make those decisions. In any case, you don't want such decisions left up to whoever is on duty at the hospital or hospice where she is receiving care, and you don't want to have to go to court to win the authority when a simple document grants those powers.

To ensure that your wife's wishes are legally guaranteed, she needs to grant someone a durable power of attorney for healthcare decisions and have a living will. With a power of attorney, your wife grants someone the power to make medical decisions if she becomes mentally incapacitated. With a living will, her exact wishes for care are spelled out. A living will mainly deal with situations surrounding the prolonging of life and covers treatments such as cardiac resuscitation and the use of feeding tubes. The document allows you to specify the treatments you want—and, just as important, the ones you do not want. You can find fill-in-the-blank versions of both documents online, but some states don't recognize such forms as legally binding. So either thoroughly research the use of online forms in your state (and don't forget that they need to be signed in front of witnesses and may also require a notary's signature) or contact a lawyer in your state who routinely handles such contracts. Do not just sign a standard form to check off a box. These are critically important documents, and I would urge you to take your time, consider their contents carefully, and make modifications as desired so that they are customized to the grantor's exact wishes.

And, of course, your wife should have a basic will that covers everything from funeral arrangements to the disposition of assets, financial and otherwise. She may want some of her keepsakes to go to particular members of the family, for example. Wills and Living wills are especially important if you are in a second marriage and one or both spouses have children from a former marriage, as Michelle did.

⸺∞⸺

Healthcare Power of Attorney

Here are highlights of what's contained in a healthcare power of attorney, as suggested by the American Bar Association:

- The person to whom I grant the right can agree to, refuse, or withdraw consent to any type of medical care, treatment, surgical procedures, tests, or medications.
- The person's authority includes decisions about using mechanical or other procedures that affect any bodily function, such as artificial respiration, artificially supplied nutrition and hydration (that is, tube feeding), cardiopulmonary resuscitation, or other forms of medical support, even if deciding to stop or withhold treatment could or would result in death.
- The person can have access to medical records and information to the same extent that I am entitled to, including the right to disclose health information to others.
- The person can authorize my admission to or discharge (even against medical advice) from any hospital, nursing home, or residential care, assisted-living or similar facility or service.
- The person can decide about organ and tissue donations, autopsy, and the disposition of my remains as the law permits.

⸺∞⸺

Working With Your Employer

Nothing is more important than being with the one you love during her time of need—not even your job. So you must use all your employer's benefits during this time. I encourage future widowers to be candid with their employer about their situation—management never likes surprises. Graciously accept what support they can offer and focus on your ailing spouse. If your employer is not supportive, and you want to take a new job, don't do so until you know how your benefits will work during the transition period to a new employer. Should you elect to change employers—and in the process, your healthcare provider—you may have a healthcare transition period during which you may have to pay medical expenses out of pocket, so be careful.

Beyond the largesse of your employer, you have rights when it comes to your job. Federal and state labor laws have provisions for family leave when employees are facing certain life events. Further, some companies—or union contracts—offer benefits that go beyond what federal and state laws may require. Using these benefits isn't a sign of weakness. These rights also benefit employers: They help employers keep their workers by providing them a reprieve when times are tough, and the workers can't focus entirely on their jobs. And taking advantage of these benefits can give you needed time to grieve while taking care of family affairs. Be sure you are familiar with your legal rights. The cornerstone of these benefits is the Family and Medical Leave Act, which requires certain employers to provide eligible employees job-protected unpaid leave (up to 12 weeks in a 12-month period) for "specified family and medical reasons including the birth, adoption or placement of a child, *care of a family member with a serious health condition*, or the employee's own serious health condition." The FMLA has additional provisions for military personnel and their families. Be sure to discuss benefits with your human resource department.

But not everyone is covered. Workers are eligible if they have been employed for at least 12 months by their employer and have worked at least 1,250 hours during the past 12 months (roughly equivalent to 25 hours per week). However, employees who meet these conditions are not eligible if their employer has fewer than 50 employees (either at the employee's worksite or within a 75-mile radius of that site). Also, if a husband and wife have the same employer, the total number of workweeks of leave to which both may be entitled could be limited to 12 if the employer so chooses.

If you make too much money in your position, you can get benefits, but your position may not be guaranteed. Such "highly compensated employees" are generally defined as salaried and being "among the highest-paid 10% of the employees." These employees are eligible for leave, but their employers are not required to restore them to their original position (or an equivalent position with equivalent pay and benefits, as is guaranteed to other employees).

While some employers don't have to pay those on family leave under the FMLA, some do. Working for such companies is a real blessing when a family crisis strikes. If your firm is not among those who are required to pay those on leave, it doesn't hurt to ask if they'll pay a portion of your wages, or make some other accommodation. Be proactive and ask what additional benefits your employer may provide. Just remember that these benefits don't just protect the worker, they help your company keep a highly valuable employee: you.

While these laws and benefits often are on the books, don't rely on your employer to suggest that you take leave under FMLA. Investigate your rights with your company's human resources department and request the benefits to which you are entitled. You may also find information available via your state department of labor's website or the FMLA Internet site: www.dol.gov/whd/fmla.

A good example of relief employers may provide *outside* of those required under Family and Medical Leave Act occurred when one of my former employers, Bank of America, provided my family with the services of a health insurance advocate. From that day forward, I never had to handle another insurance claim requested by the many healthcare providers that treated Michelle. Not having to deal with the years of claims (totaling over $1.6 million) helped me focus on Michelle's care and my duties at the bank.

You should make sure that all of your benefits remain intact if you are on FMLA leave while caring for your spouse or as you grieve following her death. Depending on the benefit, your employer may have the discretion to prorate benefits such as bonuses, vacations, and profit-sharing plans. Also, you should ask if you lose eligibility to receive annual merit increases if you are away, even for part of the year.

If your benefits are not guaranteed, you may wish to try to negotiate some consideration with management before beginning any caregiver leave period or family leave under FMLA as suggested above. Managers at your firm may have the discretion to reward valued employees extra assistance in addition to what is available under FMLA.

We need to remember that people run companies, and people differ in their compassion. Some will display great empathy; others will not. Some may even view your hardship as a means to an end so that they can give your job to someone else. I'd like to think such people are few and far between, but, hey, this is the real world.

You want your employer on your side during the difficult days ahead. It has been my experience that most companies are generous with the support they offer employees in crisis. This is particularly the case when an employee tries hard to minimize the effect of their absence. Be candid and as fair to your employer as you can be. Avoid taking advantage of your situation—for instance, by taking more time off work than you truly need. Believe me when I say that your employer—and your colleagues—will not only appreciate your team spirit but also remember your honorable conduct.

For workers who are fired or who quit their jobs to care for their wives, one option is unemployment insurance (UI), but it is not available to all. UI is a federal-state social insurance program that provides weekly benefits based on your previous earnings for up to six months, paid through employer-paid taxes. Although details vary across states, some general concepts apply. Many conditions must be met before one can receive UI. For further information, see http://www.dol.gov/dol/topic/unemployment-insurance/index.htm

Depending on his age, a widower may have one more thing going for him. He may be counted as part of a "protected class." A member of a protected class has special protections against discrimination. The Age Discrimination in Employment Act (ADEA) forbids employment discrimination against anyone at least 40 years of age in the United States. As a result of this law, employers are hard-pressed to make career matters difficult for older workers. And it's worth noting that some states have additional statutes that protect workers over 40 from age discrimination, so depending on your age, you may want to become familiar with your state's regulations from your state's labor department website or see someone in your company's employment office.

If you feel you have been treated unfairly under the provisions of the ADEA, contact your local office of the Equal Employment Opportunity Commission.

Visit the Sick

As a practicing Catholic, I was taught the seven Corporal Works of Mercy, one of which is to visit the sick. Family members and friends should be encouraged to visit seriously ill people, even if it is difficult for them. Michelle's mother and two sisters came to visit Michelle in San Antonio during the weeks before she died.

Says Dr. Carr: "Not everyone is comfortable with death. That's not an excuse for not visiting the ill, but some people worry that they will say or do the wrong thing. Confronting death head-on may be more than they can deal with."

Widower Phil Carbone says, "One of the things Lisa said shortly after her surgery was that she only wanted people around her who were upbeat and positive. As we were fortunate to have a large family and a circle of close friends, I spoke with each of them before they visited to reinforce Lisa's desire for 'positive vibes.' It worked in almost all cases. People showed their concern, but brought with them laughter, wonderful happy memories and an approach of being alive today, rather than focusing on tomorrow's procedure or the next step in her treatment."

The final days before death are especially traumatic, of course. Widower Rod Hagen said his lifetime partner, Larry, was fearful. "I had never seen him so afraid, fearing I was going to send him away to a hospital or some other kind of facility. He wanted to go to a hospice." Rod had his own fears. "I had never lived alone. I moved from my parents' house into Larry's. Before Larry died, I had done the laundry maybe three times in my entire life. I didn't talk with my friends about my deeper fear—the idea of just being alone."

Rod was raised a Protestant while Larry was raised Catholic; Larry sometimes jokingly referred to himself as a "recovering Catholic." During Larry's final days, Rod arranged for a priest to visit several times to pray with him, and to administer Larry's last rites. "Larry's and my contact with the Catholic Church was not what we expected. It was pretty amazing and supportive, while fully acknowledging our relationship."

Your Children

Finally, as I mentioned earlier, it's a good idea to enlist children in your wife's care, which will help them as well as you and your wife. And of course, older children should be told exactly what kind of illness their mother is suffering from. But according to the American Cancer Society, all children need to know specifics such as the specific name of the illness, how it will be treated, the part of the body affected, and how their own lives will be affected. Knowing these things, studies have shown, will reduce children's anxiety. So while we may want to protect them as much as possible, we can make dealing with their mother's illness more difficult if we try to shield them from the truth.

CHAPTER 2

Working Through Grief

During the weeks and months that followed Michelle's death, I knew a degree of sadness was a given, but it was far worse than I expected. I quickly saw how poorly prepared I was to deal with this grief and my new role as a widower, and how poorly prepared the world around me was to help me with either.

During my grief, I behaved like a typical man and figured I could fix what was broken. I approached widowhood as if it were my new job. I drew up lists, set priorities, and made a budget. But I wouldn't be able to delegate this problem to a junior staff member or a vendor. This widower business was mine alone to deal with. I needed to find some new tools and train myself for recovery and to realize that new challenges could arrive at my doorstep any day.

In this chapter, I'll talk about what grief is and what to expect as you grieve. I'll shed some light on how men grieve differently than women. I'll pass along advice on recovery from professionals, other widowers, and my own experience. Hopefully, this will make moving through the grieving process easier and help you avoid going down dead-end paths. I wish I had known many of these things when I was grieving over Michelle. But there are no shortcuts if you're to emerge from grief in the best shape possible: moving forward with your pain gone, or at least reduced to an ache and with the good memories of your late wife intact.

What Is Grief?

British psychiatrist Colin Murray Parkes, one of the world's leading experts on grief and the author of many books and articles on the subject, summarized grief this way: "Grief is the price for love." This quote not only rings true and has a certain poetry about it, but it is also an expert summary of the changes our brains go through when we lose love.

When we meet and fall in love, and when that love deepens over the years, our brains are wonderfully rewired. That relationship brings us joy, happiness, and comfort. It makes us feel safe and secure. And the love and the relationship are the product of two minds. Our mate does things that generate all those good feelings in us; we reciprocate, and those feelings are magnified between us. You've heard the expression, "love is a drug?" It literally is. Those feelings are the result of the release of feel-good hormones in our brains, and the deeper the relationship, the deeper our brains become wired to access those wonderful feelings in new and different ways.

That sounds a little clinical, but the bottom line is love does wonderful things for us.

Then, with the loss, the wiring that leads to so many good feelings becomes a series of paths to pain. All the great feelings and feel-good hormones now become sadness and stress hormones. In other words, when you feel grief you're paying the piper for the loss of love. It seems unfair, and it is. But grief also spurs us to seek new sources of happiness in our lives, so in that sense grief serves a useful purpose. So in our journey to recovery, think of grief and other emotions as our personal compasses pointing us to what we need to move forward.

You may have read or heard that after a loss people go through a sequence of orderly steps to recovery. The famous Kübler-Ross model, or the five stages of grief, says that, in order, we go through denial, anger, bargaining, depression and acceptance. As men, such an orderly, logical pathway sounds appealing. But while these stages have become dogma in popular culture, psychiatrist Elisabeth Kübler-Ross herself said these stages "were never meant to help tuck messy emotions into neat packages. They are responses to loss that many people have, but there is not a typical response to loss, as there is no typical loss. Our grieving is as individual as our lives."

In fact, these stages can come in different order, and some will be skipped altogether.

Widowers vary tremendously in the amount of emotional pain they experience, and how long it lasts. One widower may be grief-stricken, consumed with sorrow, broken-hearted and distressed, while another may have an easier transition.

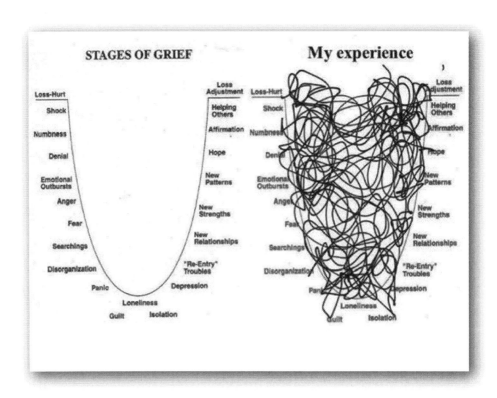

Rutgers University sociology professor Deborah Carr says that although these stages are not supported by scientific research, they may provide some comfort to those who look forward to achieving acceptance and hope in their future. In any case, Dr. Carr says, we shouldn't put expectations on widowers—there's no timetable for how long you should grieve, or even how intensely you should grieve.

Widower Steve Marquardt says well-meaning friends and family may try to typecast you as being in a specific stage. They're trying to be helpful, he says, but "it all comes down to how you feel and how you deal with things. People will try to tell you that you *need* to go through different stages of grieving. Well, maybe some people do, but you're your own best guide."

That some people think they know where your head's at in your recovery, and figure they can push you along, became apparent to me quickly. Shortly after I returned to work (just ten days after Michelle's death), a colleague offered to set me up with her aunt. I thought this woman has got to be kidding. Does she even have a clue? I responded, "That isn't going to happen," and walked away. In retrospect, I should have said, "Sure. Maybe our first date can be next week at Michelle's memorial service."

As Kübler-Ross herself said, there "is no typical loss." And in the case of us widowers, I believe the degree and quality of grief is related to what you lose when your wife dies. Your wife may have been your soulmate, and you couldn't imagine spending a day apart. Or you may have kept largely separate and independent lives. Some relationships are marked by passion, others by a warm friendship and others by a coolness that develops after years of a strained marriage. So it's not surprising that a widower's grief follows no predictable path.

How Men Grieve

But while there is no simple roadmap for grieving, there is a first step you need to take: acknowledge your grief. And science backs this up. Suppressing or denying any negative emotion can be exhausting and counterproductive, and it can create a wedge between widowers and the family members who love them. And keep in mind, Dr. Carr says, that no two people are likely to experience grief in the same way. It may take many forms—anger, guilt, irritability, social withdrawal, sleeplessness, crying, loneliness—at different times in the process. But she adds that by putting on the façade and saying, "I'm fine; don't worry about me," grieving men may be denying themselves the help they need and may find that these bottled-up feelings spill over when they least expect.

Instead of denying those feelings, own them. You can work through them if you allow yourself to experience them. Dr. Ronald G. Petrie writes in his book, *Into the Cave: When Men Grieve*, how "the only way that you become well and healed when grieving is to embrace your grief, to realize that it is a process you need to go through." Unfortunately, he says, some men refuse to take that approach, "but rather try to forget the person that they have lost. They do this by not talking about the person or trying to do anything that would remind them of the person."

Dr. Petrie, himself a widower, tells us, "Women are allowed, and in fact encouraged, to share their emotions openly within our society. Men are not."

The idea that men and women grieve differently is the main theme of the book *Grieving Beyond Gender: Understanding the Ways Men and Women Mourn*, by Kenneth Doka and Terry Martin. In reviewing this important book for the academic journal *Psychology of Women Quarterly* (February 21, 2012), Dr. Carr wrote, "Most clinicians presume that there is one most effective way to grieve. This approach typically entails a high level of emotional expression, including crying, talking out one's feeling, and relying on the emotional support of friends and professionals—in other words, a typically 'female' response to loss." In the review, Dr. Carr said that a stereotypically masculine response, "such as intellectualizing the loss or throwing one's self into work," has long been considered harmful.

As Dr. Carr told me, these are precisely the reasons why the death of a spouse can be more difficult for men than women, and an important reason why widowers are more likely than widows to die following the loss of their spouse. They bottle up their feelings and don't reach out for the help they need, sometimes desperately. Practitioners agree with this assessment. Rev. Gregg Elliott commented on his experience consoling widowers: "Men have a hard time asking for help. Men have always been taught that regardless of the situation they should be slow to ask for support. I have found this to be especially true among men with military backgrounds, as they are taught to be self-sufficient."

Dr. Phyllis R. Silverman and Scott Campbell, authors of *When Men Are Left Alone*, write: "Men mourn differently than women. They are less expressive, often very reticent, and this submerging of emotions can be harmful, physically as well as psychologically. Their feelings can range from despair and rage to a hollow sense of having no purpose."

And here's a bombshell fact to consider, and something we need to own: Emotionally, we men generally depend more on our wives then they depend on us. So as widowers we may need *more* emotional support than widows. Says Dr. Justin Denney, a sociologist at Rice University: "We have known for some time that men receive a disproportionate amount of emotional support and security from their wives. But we also expect men to be emotionally resilient or unemotional altogether. Ironically, much of the emotional strength men display in the workplace, and other realms comes from the support they receive at home. Then suddenly that support is gone, but the expectations of masculinity do not disappear along with their loved one."

Dr. Carr agrees: "In general, men need women more than the reverse. Most men don't have a whole pool of male friends with whom they feel comfortable sharing their grief. Frequently, it is their deceased wife who would have served as their confidante. The wife is also the one who makes the social plans, who sends out the holiday cards to the children. And that's why the wife is called the *kin keeper*, meaning the wife is the one who keeps the family together. Wives also keep husbands healthy."

And we men tend to focus on more tangible ways of dealing with our grief. "Men may spend more time around gravesites, tending them as a sign of their grief rather than talking or crying," says Dr. Carr. "A concrete project, like tending to a wife's grave or pulling together a memory book, may be a way for men to work through their grief in a way they are comfortable with." I guess you could say my forming the Michelle's Angels Foundation was a concrete project I took on to deal with my grief.

Ways to Cope

How we cope with this torrent of bad emotions varies greatly. I've seen all kinds of coping methods, and I know that widowers should adopt an approach they're comfortable with. Goal-oriented widowers could take the time to write down how they feel so they can see their progress, as well as identify triggers that might heighten their sadness. Widowers who prefer to express their emotions out loud or to others should be uninhibited about voicing their feelings. In fact, even screaming can be a normal part of the grieving process for some. Missing someone dear hurts. Widower John Von Der Haar shared with us how "neither Mary (his late wife) nor I ever cried very much. But after her passing, I couldn't control my tears. I yelled many times, 'Why? Why? Why?' "

Says clinical psychologist Ed Zimmer: "You could be in the middle of doing something, feeling totally okay when something unexpected triggers feelings of grief. Expect this to happen from time to time, and accept it when it does." He recommends that, "If you can, stop what you're doing and take the time to process it *in* the moment." Widower Rob Hagen tells us how one day, about one year after his partner Larry had died, he experienced a "tsunami of grief, much like what I experienced immediately after Larry had died. I was on my knees crying, going through a total meltdown and I couldn't understand why it happened."

I wish I'd known this when I lost Michelle. I was not prepared for grieving, so it's not surprising that I wasn't very good at it. I also wish I'd known that it's common to feel lost; I couldn't see a way out. Says Elizabeth Gilbert, in her soul-searching book, *Eat, Pay, Love*: "When you are standing in that forest of sorrow, you cannot imagine that you could ever find your way to a better place. But if someone can assure you that they have stood in that same place and now have moved on, sometimes this will bring hope." And I'm here to tell you that not only did I find a way through my grief, but I've interviewed dozens of widowers with different types of relationships who made it through on various paths.

In my case, following Michelle's death, I wasn't in the mood to be social, which was uncharacteristic. I was comfortable in virtually any social situation. But now I was a loner. I tried to fill my empty hours with work, so my life slid into an endless marathon of fifteen-hour days. I would arrive at Farm Bureau Bank's corporate headquarters between 4 a.m. and 5 a.m. each morning and leave at about 7 p.m. I'd have a quick dinner, perhaps watch the news and then go to bed, alone.

At one point my brother-in-law, Kent Winship, flew to San Antonio to spend some time with me and to make sure I was okay. Friends had invited the two of us to a party along the path of San Antonio's Annual Cinco de Mayo Festival Parade. Within ten minutes of my arrival, I looked at Kent and said, "I don't want to be here." I was not ready to party. I needed to be alone with my thoughts, which is natural for many of us. Yes, I appreciated those who wanted to lift my spirits, but I wasn't ready to be comforted.

Following the death of his wife, Mary, widower John Heffernan says he was in a professional fog for a long time. "It was hard for me to concentrate and equally hard for me to focus and remember simple things that I would have easily remembered before. Life was a blur. But it was important for me to get up and out of the house every day and *go to work*. This work routine established some purpose for me."

This "fog" isn't surprising. Dr. Carr, author of *Worried Sick: How Stress Hurts Us and How to Bounce Back*, says that grief reactions aren't just emotional; they can cause cognitive impairments as well. When our stress levels are high, as they are in the aftermath of a major loss, dopamine (or the "pleasure hormone") levels are affected in ways that impede our memory and concentration.

For some widowers, like John, their poor work focus reflected that. John explains: "I quickly recognized that Mary was my motivation for making money and being successful. I found myself being a bit sloppy in my business dealings and not being as driven as I was when Mary was there to impress. There was a silver lining for John, though. He says, "I've settled into a simple business routine and have given up on conquering the world. I spend more time working to understand problems of others and helping them find solutions. I'm less focused on financial success and much more focused on my personal relationships."

Widows and widowers find many different ways to cope with loss. While women tend to reach out to friends for emotional support, men often seek out activities to help them manage their grief or serve the memory of their late wives. Dr. Carr explains that coping behaviors can be classified as "emotion-focused," which are ones that work to sooth one's feelings, or "problem-focused," which are behaviors that are action-oriented to distract or otherwise engage oneself during times of distress. In general, women tend to use emotion-focused strategies whereas men tend to adopt more problem-focused approaches.

Dealing With Guilt and Regret

As if grief weren't bad enough, often guilt is associated with grieving, and we need to understand this strong emotion as well. We typically feel it when we think we haven't lived up to some moral standard.

It's no surprise that some widowers—especially those who feel they didn't do all they could do as caregivers and husbands—may experience powerful feelings of guilt. "It's inevitable that some widowers might feel guilty," say Dr. Carr. "Spouses are expected to care for each other, in sickness and health, until death do they part. It's difficult to recognize that hard work and love were not enough to sustain a spouse's life." She adds that feelings of guilt can be magnified given that caregiving now more often takes place at home so that husbands may take on a greater role taking care of their wives. As more aspects of care fall to family members, these deputized caregivers may feel that they were ill-prepared and could have made a mistake administering medications, for example. "It is not surprising, then, that even caregivers who have done all they could still feel guilty."

That includes me. Following Michelle's death, I couldn't help but relive the decisions I made related to her care over and over. Were they the right choices? Were they truly in her best interest, or was I trying to balance her needs with mine? Did I compromise when better options were available? Did I comfort her enough? Was moving to San Antonio a mistake?

Widower John Von Der Haar says, "I have immense feelings of guilt. Did I get the right treatment for her? Should we have used more aggressive treatments? There are a lot of things that I regret, and a lot of things that I would have done differently. There are a lot of things that I should have said that I didn't."

Regret is a close cousin to guilt, and widower regrets can be sparked for many reasons. Says Steve Marquardt about his time with his wife Merethe during her illness: "I definitely would have spent much more time with her." But Steve shouldn't beat himself up too much. He and Merethe were a one-income family, so Steve needed to work to provide for their two children and Merethe's daughter Amy. But even with this, given my own experience, I completely understand the regret of not spending enough time with an ailing wife.

Widower Aaron Seiden is a remarkable man from Baltimore, Maryland, who at the age of 18 went ashore at Normandy as part of the invasion of Europe. Aaron told me how after he was shot twice, he never thought he would reach the age of 19, let alone his age of 90. Aaron says that one of the great regrets of his long life is how he should have told his wife he loved her more often. Aaron encourages all husbands: "Tell your wife several times each day how much you love her."

Widower and Pastor Bob Page remembers, "My wife always wanted to dance, and I wouldn't dance with her. And now I live in The Villages, a residential community in Florida where people dance every night. I regret not granting her wish. I was simply too stuffy."

So how do you get past feelings of guilt and regret? The key is to forgive yourself, which isn't as easy as it sounds. You'll need to fess up to your shortcomings honestly. You will need to learn from those shortcomings and change your moral code so that you won't repeat them. Then you'll need to stick to that code. Once that's done, you can put those feelings behind you.

Reaching for Help

As I said at the beginning of this chapter, grief means we've been cut off from a relationship that brought us all kinds of emotional benefits. Part of our recovery is finding sources of emotional support that will help assuage the sting of that loss.

For us men, that's often a tough thing to do. This was driven home to me in the spring of 2014 when a friend of mine, retired minister Paul Hubley, arranged for me to meet with a group of widowers, each a resident of the Elim Park facility in Cheshire, Connecticut. After speaking to the gathering of widowers about my loss and trials, I was amazed how engaged the men became. The men shared stories, and tears flowed as each man recounted his loss and the pain he had carried—for many of these men, it was the first time they had spoken of their feelings, and it was obvious they felt better for sharing them with other widowers. It was one of the most moving experiences I had while working on this book.

On my trip home, it hit me that widowers need permission to grieve and to share. Today, most do not feel they have permission, or they fear that others will think less of them as a man if they expose their grief. For that single reason, one widower I spoke with decided not to participate in this book. He was afraid that once he revealed his story and his emotions, others would see him as weak.

I admit that I didn't reach out as soon as I should have for all the support and fellowship I needed. I recall one day, as I worked at my desk at the bank, one of the employees from the bank's call center entered my office with her brow furrowed by concern. She quietly told me how "everyone on the floor misses your laughter." That helped me see myself from a different vantage, and thanks to that caring soul I began to realize that I was not in a good place physically or emotionally. I realized I needed help, and I resolved to find it.

Men don't need to go it alone. Those who have friends and family should reach out to them. For those who don't have loved ones nearby or who don't feel comfortable asking friends and family for assistance, there are other services available. Hospice, which provides comfort care and support to dying patients, also can be an important source of support and empathy for caregiving husbands and widowers. For instance, hospice offered widower Rod Hagen counseling for one year following the loss of his partner, Larry. Every ten days or so, the same man would call Rod, so he had someone to speak with—someone who understood what he was going through. Rod added, "The hospice volunteer ended up calling me for nearly two years. I wasn't asked to come to some meeting and sit with a group of strangers and talk about my loss. Hospice was great. I also had a couple of close friends who were there when I needed to talk, and even when I didn't need to talk but I didn't want to be alone."

Widowers need a support network. I refer to them as a widower's Personal Advisory Board. They could be a team hailing from your collection of lifelong friends, neighbors, a fellow congregant from your religious community, relatives, or a select group of professionals (doctor, lawyer, financial planner, life-coach, etc.). Your Personal Advisory Board represents your *go-to* team, the ones you should make familiar with your life situation and allow to advise you as needed. Forming a Personal Advisory Board is a great way to allow another person who is also grieving over the loss of your wife to offer their support. You could even say it would be therapeutic for both of you.

Fellowship with other widowers through a widower group, or even with just a single widower, can be a valuable part of your Personal Advisory Board. Widower Chris Sweet tells us how he reached out and found one of his old high school buddies who had also lost his wife. "He and I used to play basketball together but lost touch after graduation. When his wife died, I felt horrible for him. I remember how I didn't know what to say to him. After some time, I found myself thinking how, given his loss, he was aware of what I was going through, and might be able to help me make sense out of what was going on with me. We spoke on the phone and exchanged e-mails. That was what I needed to keep me going."

Check for widower support groups at local churches, hospitals, and hospices. Or you may want to check out groups through www.nationalwidowers.org. Let me also invite you to register with the Widower's Support Network, which I founded. Its mission is to comfort and assist widowers by offering free services. See www.WidowersSupportNetwork.com. Other resources that might be of help to widowers include www.onetoanother.org, a service that enables men and women who have experienced loss to meet, and www.widowedvillage.org, which connects widows and widowers for friendship and sharing.

In my research, I also discovered that a pet can be a great source of comfort during a time of grief. After personally witnessing the effect that animals can have, I became a believer. But rather than go into that here—I know pets are not for everyone—I've written up my research in Appendix III.

No Grief and Perpetual Grief

Sometimes widowers experience no grief after the death of their spouse. The reasons for this vary. During my research for this book, I met some men who quietly celebrated what they considered their emancipation from an imperfect marriage. But such cases were rare.

Some men go through many stages of grief while their wife is still alive—especially if a wife's illness was long and difficult. Says widower Jeff Gower: "I can remember how some people thought I was really calm the first 24 hours following Susan's death. Well, Susan had been dying for five years, and I'd been dying with her for five years."

Dr. Carr says that "all marriages are different, and we never know what goes on behind closed doors. An unhappy spouse shouldn't be judged for not grieving the loss of a wife, whereas a widower who had a close relationship shouldn't feel that he's not coping well." Carr notes that grief often is not the primary emotion that widowers feel when their wife dies following a long and painful illness. Rather, they may feel relief—and they shouldn't feel guilty about that. "For men who provided care to their dying wives, and who watched them suffer for months if not years, death brings a peaceful close to their suffering. Men should not feel guilty if their wife's death brings them a sense of relief in knowing that she is out of her pain and now at peace."

At the other end of the grief spectrum is grief that seems never ending. The process of grief takes time, says clinical psychologist

Edward Zimmer, and that time varies from man to man. But over time, men should gradually return to the activities and habits they had before their loss. Zimmer suggests that the one-year mark should be a time of self-reflection to gauge your recovery. And he says that if a widower has not returned to most of his pre-loss activities after a year to 18 months, which may be evidence of not moving through the grief process.

Men who are still experiencing severe grief symptoms may suffer from what clinicians call complicated grief. This entails feelings of acute grief; a preoccupation with thoughts of the deceased; an inability to re-establish daily routines; turning away from friends and family, and avoiding things that once gave pleasure. Complicated grief strikes only 7% of bereaved people, according to Columbia University researcher M. Katherine Shear. But if you have these symptoms, it's time to consult a psychologist, psychiatrist or other medical professional.

To recap, there's no one way to grieve the loss of a spouse. But we need to face that grief, find strategies that work best for us, and find people who can provide us with emotional support and counsel. By using grief and other emotions as a compass, together with patience and persistence, we can move through grief on our journey to recovery.

Here are some additional resources you may want to try:

GriefShare (www.GriefShare.org). GriefShare is a website that will put you in touch with people so that you don't have to go through one of life's most painful experiences alone.

Grief Recovery Institute (www.griefrecoverymethod.com). Offers support via its website, social media, and its counseling sessions in the U.S. and Canada, with affiliates in Sweden, the United Kingdom and most recently Mexico.

National Widowers Organization (www.nationalwidowers.org). This group "educates the public about the special needs of men who have lost their spouse or life partner." They accomplish this by "promoting the development of support groups for men to manage their grief and adjust to a new life and by advocating for research into men's unique needs to deal with grief and spousal loss."

Open to Hope (www.opentohope.com). A nonprofit foundation with the mission of helping people find hope after loss.

Recover-from-grief (www.recover-from-grief.com). A source of information for those grieving and who are seeking straight answers, practical advice, and hope.

Soaring Spirits International (www.sslf.org). Provides "innovative peer-based grief support programs for widowed men and women."

The Grief Toolbox (www.thegrieftoolbox.com). This is a resource every widower should become familiar with. Provides helpful articles, gift items, networking, and more.

Widowers Grief (www.widowersgrief.blogspot.com). Each Wednesday, host Mark Liebenow, an author of four books and a Huffington Post blogger, shares his connections with nature as a means of comforting those who grieve.

Widower's Support Network (www.WidowersSupportNetwork. com). The organization I founded has as its mission to comfort and assist widowers by offering free services.

CHAPTER 3

Restoring Your Life

As we discussed in the last chapter, grieving is the most difficult leg of our widower's journey. But we face other hurdles. Bereavement researchers Margaret Stroebe and Henk Schut say widowers and widows have two types of challenges: *loss-related* tasks, which means dealing with emotional loss, and *restoration-oriented* tasks, which means re-establishing one's daily routines and practices. We widowers handle these on parallel tracks, and usually not in sync. One day we may feel reasonably happy and at peace, but struggle with preparing a dinner for one. Another day we may take care of the bills, but feel profoundly lonely.

For widowers, restoration-oriented tasks can be more difficult than we think because we often take for granted the many things our wives did to help keep our households—and our lives in general—chugging along. For instance, widower John Heffernan told me that he was "totally unprepared to take over household finances" following the loss of his wife, Mary.

So in this chapter, we'll talk about putting your life back together. We'll cover dealing with loneliness, handling mundane tasks, rebuilding a social life, and finally finding meaning in your life, which may be lost when you lose your wife. Many widowers choose to restore their lives by finding a new romantic partner or wife. Let me suggest that doing this too quickly is a mistake and can lead to bad relationships and broken hearts. (I discuss dating in Chapter 7.) If you first work on restoring your life, you'll approach a new relationship as a whole person—not as half of a one-time couple—with more to offer.

Loneliness

Defeating loneliness is a crucial trial in your journey. And being single again often means painful bouts of loneliness, which is a pain most of us can't imagine when still married. Nearly all of us know what it's like to be alone, even when we're married. For instance, when Michelle and I were temporarily apart, say because of a business trip, I was lonely for her. But I knew we'd soon be back together. I didn't know about profound loneliness until she was gone forever. This type of loneliness is like true hunger. You can't know true hunger if you're just dieting; true hunger is starving without knowing when or if your next meal is coming.

Often, we widowers are reluctant to admit loneliness and what we miss most about our late wives. That's too bad, because knowing that others share the same pain can help ease our own. A good first step to addressing the special loneliness you feel is to speak with other widowers, as recommended in the last chapter. But barring that, I'd like to spend a few paragraphs sharing some thoughts on the subject—both my own and those of other widowers.

Day after day when I returned to a home without Michelle, I was lonely for everything—from her car parked in my space at the end of a long day to her giggle to her perfume. I went to sleep next to the empty half of the bed we had shared.

It's a common feeling. Says widower and Pastor Bob Page: "The hardest part of being alone was walking into the house. I didn't even want to drive into the garage." Widower Aaron Seiden feels that "as a widower, the worst part is the silence. I hated to come home, put the key in the lock on the door, and then be greeted by a wall of silence. I tried to remedy this by always having the TV or radio on."

Widower Harold Moran says that the absence of an intimate relationship can be unbearable. "I'm not just talking about making love, but the intimacy of cuddling at night, sharing dreams, holding hands, and planning for the future. The many things loving couples do every day to stay connected. A gentle hand on the shoulder after a hard day, a passing kiss as two souls move about during a busy day. That fun slap on her butt while she has her hands elbow deep in dishwater. It's a million things that are suddenly gone." For widower John Von Der Haar, the lack of sharing hurt the most. "There is no one to share the day's experiences—no one to share funny stories, housework, yard work, meals, coffee, walks, or anything else."

And then there are loneliness triggers, which include all the *firsts* to get past. The first Christmas without Michelle. The first New Year's Eve. The first birthday, Mother's Day, wedding anniversary, family reunion, Thanksgiving. A child's wedding. And yes, even the anniversary of her death. Feeling a special pain on such days is a common problem. Research by Rutgers University sociology professor Deborah Carr and her colleagues found that older men and women who had been recently widowed reported particularly high symptoms of sadness during the month of their late spouse's birthday.

Some widowers treat their loneliness by clinging to their wives' possessions. Dr. Carr says these "continuing bonds" can be healthy, as they provide comfort and uplifting memories. "Pictures, perfume, playing her favorite piece of music, for instance, are all perfectly healthy ways to keep a beloved wife 'present' even when her body is no longer here." However, she cautions, it isn't healthy when clinging to cherished objects from the past prevents us from engaging in the present and moving forward.

I recall that after my mother died in 1981, my father never dismantled my mother's bedroom. For years, her bottles of perfume remained on her dresser top; her clothes stayed neatly hung in her closet; all of her hats were precisely stored in boxes and placed on the top shelf. My father simply could not remove evidence of her life. I'm sure many of you understand why he felt that way.

As widower John Von Der Haar approached the three year mark since he had lost his beloved Mary, he had not yet moved anything belonging to her. "I have tried to do something with her clothes and other belongings, but can't," he told me. "I found a shirt that we had embroidered with the logo of our first sailboat in 1981 and could not take it from the hanger. Likewise, the sweatshirt from the time we visited Yosemite caught me by surprise. Because I know where and when she bought a lot of her clothing, almost every item brings back memories."

Often, men will try to cope with this void by turning to alcohol. But drinking heavily won't bring back your wife—and it may make you susceptible to depression, aggression, or even physical health problems like liver disease, obesity, and diabetes. Drinking might also limit your ability to work, keep up happy relationships with family and friends, or even pursue a new romantic relationship.

More than a few men told me they turned to the bottle in their darkest days. Harold Moran says, "I'll admit that alcohol does serve as a source of comfort. But when the morning sun comes up, nothing has changed, and I'm still alone."

Widower Phil Carbone had a similar reaction. "I was rudderless. I didn't seek a counselor, but I should have. I did increase my drinking, which of course didn't help."

Dr. Carr says that being alone and being lonely are not the same thing. Being alone simply means being by one's self. Many people are perfectly happy with their own company. Loneliness is different, and comes in two types, according to psychologists: emotional and social. Emotional loneliness refers to the absence of an intimate confidante, while social loneliness refers to the absence of a broader social network. Widowers need to figure out what loneliness they're feeling— emotional, social, or both. Emotional loneliness can be addressed by heart-to-heart conversations with a dear friend, or with a therapist to get you started. You can dip into your Personal Advisory Board, as I discussed in the last chapter, to find a confidante. Social loneliness can be helped by just being with a group of people, such as joining a book group, playing poker, or volunteering.

Managing the Mundane

Let's take a break from managing our spiritual recovery to talk about some mundane things—because, as Stroebe and Schut teach, these things are important as well.

One of the most painful jolts that we widowers feel is the realization that everyday life goes on as usual. Though our world has been turned upside down, the earth doesn't stop spinning. The tiny acts that order and thread through the day still demand our attention.

With most couples, the partners divide up tasks so that the household runs smoothly, says Dr. Carr. But when one of the partners dies, daily routines are turned upside down. After Michelle had died, I wondered, who is going to weed the garden, clean the house, call the plumber, pay the bills, and fix the meals? And, damn, I need groceries.

Widower Rutilo Flores wrote an open letter to his late wife, Raka. In it, Rutilo wrote, "You taught me so many things during the 30-plus years that I knew you and during our 25 years of marriage, but you never taught me how to live without you."

Widower Phil Carbone admits that he struggled with home-maintenance tasks after his wife died. "The home was an albatross. I resented the house, the maintenance, and the yard work." But he sought out new skills and even new passions. He says, "I found that food shopping and cooking were excellent distractions that I started to look forward to. For widowers who don't know how to cook, take some classes. You might be surprised at the escape and focus it provides."

And I would add that cooking classes are a great way to find a group to address your social loneliness.

Some men even surprised themselves with the skills they acquired. Rutilo recalled, "I never learned how to cook. Men from my country [Mexico] never enter the kitchen. Today, I am a good cook." Research by Dr. Carr shows that widows and widowers who were once highly dependent on their spouses for cooking, cleaning, and home maintenance went on to experience great gains in their self-esteem by mastering new skills and learning to live solo.

Of course, not every widower wants to become a master chef or even a passable cook. Widower Paul Dispenza was fortunate when, following the passing of his wife, Melissa, friends, and family delivered so much food to his home he didn't have to cook for months. He explained, "Those that supported us with food arranged for it using a terrific website called Take Them a Meal." The site (www.takethemameal.com) is a free service that lets family and friends coordinate food deliveries.

Rebuilding a Social Life

There comes a time when a widower must re-enter the social world. As a new widower, I found that some social occasions, such as dinners and dances, could be awkward because I stood out. You've been a husband, and suddenly you're a single. I was envious of couples I saw walking together—or even sitting next to each other in a car as I waited for a traffic light to change.

And worse than those awkward moments is how you may lose friends when you become a widower. That, I learned, is something many of my fellow widowers dealt with. Unfortunately, several of the couples Michelle and I had befriended disappeared from my life. In some cases, I'm sure it was because Michelle was the glue that held the relationships together. I know I missed our old friends, but I didn't want to chase relationships that I thought were not mutually valued.

But sometimes widowers are left out in the cold because our friends—especially our married friends—simply don't know what to say or do around us. We make them uncomfortable. It may be because our presence reminds them of the death of someone they also loved, or even that we remind them of their own mortality. Dr. Carr says widowers and widows often lament that they feel abandoned by their friends. "Rarely is this abandonment rooted in malicious intent. Rather, death makes people uncomfortable, and even long-time friends don't know what to say to a widow or widower. They're afraid of saying the wrong thing, of hurting us. Yet others don't want to see a living, breathing reminder that life is finite."

Dr. Carr says: "The importance of social support cannot be overstated; for widowhood as well as many other stressors we face in life, having a confidante—even just one close friend—can do a world of good. Both close-knit friendships and confidantes can be useful for heart-to-heart talks, but we also benefit from more-casual acquaintances that are just fun. These can be clubs, men's groups, sports teams, and the like."

You don't have to jump in with both feet, and in any case, you may not feel ready to. I know I eased in, but each step was an important one I still remember. For example, five months after Michelle died, my stepson, Jacques, and I went to a minor league baseball game with my colleagues from Farm Bureau Bank.

But such steps can be surprisingly tough for many of us, especially if we didn't have much social contact outside of what we did with our wives, or we're naturally shy, or if we're depressed. And at first, social outings may even generate more stress for us, or increase feelings of loneliness until we're accepted into a new social circle.

But not only are activities great for social contact, they can also be a great way to establish a new identity or rediscover an old identity that might have been put on the shelf while you were caring for your dying wife. For instance, widower Keith Merriam got back into the Society for Creative Anachronism, an international history group that studies and recreates Medieval European cultures and their histories. Keith also sought out and joined a community theater group. If you enjoy painting, take an art class. Love to read? Join a book group. Athletic? Get in a softball or basketball league.

Finding New Relevance

As I said at the start of this chapter, many widowers rush into a new relationship to fill the void in their lives. I get that. It's a quick way to address your loneliness, rebuild a social life, and even handle life's mundane challenges. With a new relationship, you're no longer a half of a whole; you've found a new half to make you whole.

But let's look at the issue of our loss from another perspective. Part of your identity as a husband was probably as a provider and, if your wife had a long illness, as a caretaker. Such things give us relevance in life, just as our careers do, and just as being a father does. The loss of a wife can cause a loss of relevance. In this final section, I'd like to discuss regaining or strengthening your relevance as a part of helping to restore your life. For me, as I've mentioned, I started the not-for-profit, Michelle's Angels Foundation, Inc., to help those in need.

Professor Carr notes that people often find a new sense of purpose or mission in life after a loved one dies. Often, the inspiration comes from trying to right the wrong that killed our loved one. Parents of children who die of overdoses dedicate themselves to teaching about the evils of drugs. Widowers whose wives died of breast cancer may walk or run in breast cancer fundraiser events in her honor and memory. These charitable activities make us feel connected to something larger than ourselves.

After Jeff Gower and his wife, Susan, learned of her diagnosis of ovarian cancer, the two of them dedicated themselves to promoting ovarian cancer awareness as volunteers. Two months after Susan's passing in 2005, someone asked Jeff if it was too soon for him to be called upon to speak to an audience about ovarian cancer, to which Jeff remarked, "It's never too early to get the word out on ovarian cancer." He has addressed many audiences since.

I met Jeff when he attended one of my speaking engagements. He says: "I came to hear Herb speak because I wanted to educate myself better on how to help other widowers. We are here for a purpose—to lead, to dance and love again. No matter what our purpose has been in the past, it might be stronger than ever following the loss of a wife. Go out and do some good. Make the world better in some way. This is why I will do all I can to help any man that has been widowed."

After Carl Jahrstorfer had lost his wife, Patricia, he created a scholarship fund for people who work at the nursing home where he's employed. It is funded by donations and by the sale of a book written by his wife, titled *Walk with Me* (for a copy, check out www. xulongpress.com). The book is a compilation of six months of e-mails that Patricia felt compelled to write while she underwent chemotherapy and surgery for ovarian cancer. It's a moving collection of personal thoughts, insights, and inspiration. The confidence with which Patricia faced her final days is remarkable. Following Patricia's passing, Carl finished writing Patricia's book and had it published.

Ray Henderson lost his wife in 2005. A resident of North Charleston, S.C., Ray was a computer programmer who was more accustomed to writing code than comforting others. But he wanted to help, so in 2011 he decided to start volunteering for the Red Cross, and the Red Cross showed him the way. Ray has been there after a fire in Myrtle Beach, to aid a community in Oklahoma that had been ravaged by a tornado, and to care for others after the devastation left by Hurricane Sandy. Men often gain a sense of accomplishment by building things. In Ray's case, he is rebuilding people's lives as well as the communities they live in. Ninety-six percent of Red Cross workers are volunteers, so if you think you would be interested in lending a hand as well as your compassion and skills, why not give them a call?

But whether by doing work for a large organization, such as the American Red Cross or the American Cancer Society, or by working on a worthwhile project for your church, you are likely to gain more in return than you may think. And if you're hesitating to volunteer because you don't believe you have the required skills, think again. Give your favorite not-for-profit a call. You'll be warmly received.

Relevance comes in many forms. One month after he lost his wife of almost 73 years, 96-year-old Fred Stobaugh, from Peoria, Illinois, wrote the lyrics to a song that he never imagined would be recorded. But by coincidence, Green Shoe Studios, a new recording studio located near Fred's home, announced a songwriting contest about the same time he wrote his song. Fred thought, Why not? So he entered the contest.

You can imagine his delight when he received a call from the studio, telling him how they were so moved by his story and song that they decided to produce it.

Oh, Sweet Lorraine was born. A heartfelt ballad that became a recording sensation, *Oh Sweet Lorraine* entered the Billboard Hot 100 at number 43 in September 2013. Fred's story exploded across the nation and around the world. To learn more about Fred's remarkable story and to hear *Oh Sweet Lorraine*, search the song title on YouTube. Sadly, just before going to print on this book, I learned how Fred had passed away and has now rejoined his Sweet Lorraine.

Just like dealing with grief, getting your life on track isn't easy and takes time. Your first challenge may be loneliness, and you may bounce between a longing for your departed spouse and struggling with mundane tasks around the house. Learning new skills and building a new social life can both address loneliness and be empowering, giving us a sense of confidence and purpose that we haven't felt in years. It isn't easy, but as I have discovered, a new happiness is out there. It just takes time and conscious engagement to find.

CHAPTER 4
Protecting Your Health

Men are naturally great at many things. For example, we're experts at making fire and cooking meat. But one thing at which we stink is taking care of ourselves. The Cleveland Clinic surveyed hundreds of American men and found that not only was health not a topic of conversation (men are five times more likely to talk about sports than their health), it was roundly ignored by most. The survey found that just three in five men get an annual physical, and a large percentage (more than 40%) go to the doctor only when they think they may have a serious medical condition. And about 1 in 5 said they go to the doctor *so their partner will stop nagging them.*

So when we experience a traumatic event, and our health falls into jeopardy because of it, we're poorly prepared. The deep sadness you're experiencing, as we've earlier noted, leads to higher rates of stress-induced disease, depression, post-traumatic stress disorder, and suicide. In this chapter, we'll help you past these risks. We'll show you the evidence, the warning signs, and the practical steps to take to recover from and to avoid health problems. And remember:

If you're not healthy—or worse, if you die—you're in no position to help family and friends who need your strength.

Warning: We're heading into some depressing territory here (and yes, we will talk about depression). But while I won't pull any punches about the physical and mental problems we face, I'll give remedies at the end of the chapter. And speaking of punches, I spoke to a lot of men who found the simple act of hitting something (no, not someone) to be therapeutic. It might be a punching bag, a racquetball, or a golf ball. It's not a cure-all, but we're men, and hitting stuff is another thing we're good at. And that's good for us.

Health and emotional recovery are closely connected, and which to address first is a bit of a chicken-or-egg challenge. The best strategy: attack them at the same time, because poor health hinders emotional recovery and vice versa. Today, whenever I speak with a caregiver or widower, I encourage them to be mindful of their own health and to see a doctor regularly. I speak from experience—specifically after two events that occurred following Michelle's passing.

The first struck hard and fast, and the second I'll talk about at the end of this chapter. Driving home after my first day back at work after Michelle's death, I discovered that I had a passenger—anxiety—that grew bigger by the mile. I tried to stay positive, but anxiety was winning. *This time our home.....my home.....will be different. The fragrance of her perfume will still be there, but I will not hear her voice greet me, see the warmth of her smile, or feel the comfort of her hug.* I pulled into the garage and suddenly felt a stabbing pain on my left side that bloomed into agony.

Fortunately, Jacques, my stepson, arrived home a few minutes later and raced me to the emergency room. Lying in the ER with doctors around me, I heard Jacques say, "I can't afford to lose two parents in two weeks." As it turned out, I had kidney stones, just ten days after Michelle's death. Doctors had to surgically remove the stones four excruciating days later. Of course, the kidney stones don't form in ten days, but I'm convinced the stress and anxiety I felt brought on the attack.

Stress-Induced Illness

The stress caregivers feel before a wife's death and the stress from grief afterward degrades their bodies. Stress increases the level of cortisol—a hormone with far-reaching effects—in our bodies. Best known as the "fight or flight" hormone, cortisol can be a good thing in the short term, says Dr. Carr. "If a predator is chasing you, cortisol levels rise, giving you the energy to run away." But living under persistent, high levels of stress, and therefore high levels of cortisol is like constantly running your car's engine above the red line. The body can't keep up the tension, high heart rate and stressed body chemistry when constantly in overdrive. "The result leaves the widower more vulnerable to falling ill," Dr. Carr says.

Dr. Anil K. Sood, from the MD Anderson Cancer Center in Houston, describes the difference between short-term and chronic stress. Short-term stress may surface on your wedding day or during a job interview. This type of stress generally disappears once the root cause has passed, he says. Chronic or long-term stress is damaging. Chronic stress comes from situations that last for extended periods with no definite end point. Caring for a sick spouse or a loved one is a common cause of chronic stress, and such stress weakens your immune system, leaving you vulnerable to disease, depression, and digestive problems.

Dr. Carr points to studies showing that of forty-five possible stressful scenarios, the death of a spouse is the most stressful experience for married people. The second-most-stressful experience also involved the loss of a spouse: Divorce.

An extreme but not uncommon case is that of Jack McCarthy. He was very much in love with his Barbara, but also dependent on her—so much so that he was unable to live without her. Jack's entire life revolved around Barbara, and her life revolved around his. From managing the home finances to setting their social calendar, Barbara guided the lives they shared. When Barbara passed away from cancer, Jack was so distraught that he lay down on a sofa and died—some believe of a *broken heart*—within twenty-seven hours of Barbara's passing, according to their son, Tim.

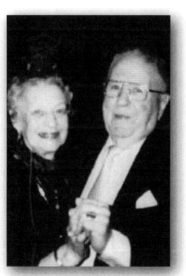

Jack (Mac) and Barbara McCarthy

Dr. Carr notes that this scenario—in which one spouse dies not long after the other—is often interpreted as a romantic tragedy: dying of a broken heart. But that's not really the case. Rather, some men are highly dependent on their wives for healthy meals, as well as reminders to take their medicine, exercise, or get a good night's sleep. When their wife dies, the health-enhancing support she provides dies with her, leaving men physically vulnerable and susceptible to illness.

These dependent men are uniquely vulnerable. Unable to deal with what may appear as even the simplest of tasks, they may consciously or subconsciously seek to find a new partner. Dr. Carr says this is exactly what her research has found: Men who had been highly reliant on their wives were much more eager to date and remarry, whereas men who were able to carry out their wives' former tasks and who had socially supportive friendships had less of a need to date and remarry.

Physical Illnesses That Can Be Caused by Stress

- High blood pressure
- Heart disease
- Stroke
- Infections from decreased immunity
- Digestive problems such as ulcers
- Cancer

Symptoms of Stress

Physical

- Elevated heart rate
- Shaking
- Problems sleeping

Psychological

- Sadness
- Loss of interest in usual activities
- Nervousness
- Inability to concentrate
- Thoughts of suicide
- Uncontrollable thoughts about the deceased or dying

Behaviors

- Inability to work
- Not caring about personal hygiene
- Increased smoking, drinking or reliance on drugs

—⚬⚬⚬—

The consequences of such stress to widowers are dire. To cite just one study led by Javier Espinosa at the Rochester Institute of Technology, men are 30% more likely to die than women soon after losing their spouse. And according to the U.S. Department of Health and Human Services, there are four times as many widows (8.7 million) as widowers (2.1 million). There's a good reason for this imbalance, according to Dr. Espinosa: "When a wife dies, men are often unprepared. They have often lost their caregiver, someone who cares for them physically and emotionally, and the loss directly affects the husband's health."

The irony is painful. The loss of a wife not only causes grief that generates health issues, the wife often was the person most responsible for helping her husband lead a healthier life. Let's be honest: We men aren't the best at getting regular health screenings, taking prescriptions, eating right, and having routine procedures such as colonoscopies or getting checked for prostate problems. In fact, when faced with a health issue, women are three times more likely to check with a doctor than men are, according to a Loyola University study.

And the neglect of our health may date back to when our wife was too ill to remind us to take care of ourselves. Dr. Carr points out that when a widower experiences a minor pain in his chest, he may think, "Oh, that's nothing compared with what my wife has to deal with," and he dismisses his symptoms.

Let's put an even finer point on this: Dr. Carr cited a Scandinavian study of several thousand widowers that found they more often suffered from diseases linked to unhealthy behaviors related to being widowers, including cirrhosis of the liver, lung cancer, diabetes, and heart attacks. The reason is their wives often helped them cut back on smoking, drinking, driving accidents, and eating unhealthy foods. "When the wife dies, her helpful reminders go with her," says Dr. Carr.

We men often don't receive the care and attention we need in part due to the traditional way American society views us. Consider that almost 3,000 people were killed in the September 11, 2001, terrorist attacks on the World Trade Center, and one-fourth of them were women—many with husbands and children. Yet the coverage following the tragedy focused almost exclusively on widows and fatherless children, with little attention given to widowers. A 2002 article in the *Boston Globe* asked, "So why the imbalance?" One answer in the story was: "American culture is uncomfortable with male grief." The *Globe* wrote: "There is no getting around that [in media coverage about 9/11] widowers are dramatically less visible than their female counterparts. Widows may outnumber widowers five to one, but the national media coverage has to be ten times as skewed." Commenting in the article, grief therapist Elizabeth Levang, author of *When Men Grieve: Why Men Grieve Differently and How You Can*

Help (Fairview Press, 1998), noted how men are "responsible for managing the family grief." To be strong for their families, she said, "these men maintain outward stoicism, mourning only sporadically and in solitude."

And again, that emotional repression causes the type of stress that is so damaging. I can also attest that widowed men differ greatly in their ability to handle stress. Some have experience handling stress and have developed coping skills, and some are just wired better to withstand it. But others lack the support of family and friends or the financial resources to get professional help.

Before we get to the subject of depression, let's discuss suppression. Emotional suppression is a root cause of many medical issues suffered by widowers, including depression. And suppression is something we men excel at and are even trained to do while we're growing up. Bridget Webber, an Australian clinical psychologist, warns, "When emotions are held back or suppressed consistently, people are liable to hurt themselves."

Clinical psychologist Edward Zimmer adds: "Some widowers underestimate the importance of expressing strong emotion and handle their grief by suppressing feelings they're aware of. Whether the acknowledgment of feelings is consciously suppressed or unconsciously repressed, both can lead to physical symptoms. They may also lead to mood symptoms such as unexpected anger, depression or guilt, or behaviors such as substance abuse."

Depression

Winston Churchill called it his "black dog." Abraham Lincoln said it made him feel like "the most miserable man living." Even Sigmund Freud battled it, with cocaine (unsuccessfully). Few widowers are likely to escape suffering some depression.

A few weeks after Michelle passed away, the stress pushed me into depression. Thankfully, one day my sister Sandy called to check up on me. Being a nurse, she asked some questions and quickly realized I wasn't coping well. She suggested I see a doctor and even suggested that the doctor may want to prescribe antidepressants. I took her advice, and I'm glad I did. I only needed the medication for a month, but it made a big difference in lessening my depression. I know I got off easy. Depression can last for months or years. The antidepressants not only elevated my mood but also let me think more clearly and prevented the dark thoughts swirling around in my head from overwhelming me.

Widower Harold Moran said he was constantly dogged by depression. "Even though I tried to remain optimistic, I had this feeling that I was losing it as I experienced mood swings and bouts of depression." Harold's brother Earnest, who is also a double widower, tells us: "I didn't know what I needed, or if I even wanted to stop the hurt. I felt if I did, I would be disloyal to my wife. Besides, the pain was all I had left."

It's hard for those who have never experienced deep depression to understand that it can be a state that becomes normal, even desirable. Several of this book's contributing widowers have offered similar views, even describing their state of misery as becoming comfortable.

According to Dr. Carr, evolutionary scholars have shown how short-term depression can be *good* for us. "For men, in particular, depression signals to others that help is needed. Signals include if a widower's personality changes, a sluggish walk, unkempt clothing, missing meetings, or not leaving his house. People need to respond to these not-so-subtle cues that the widower is struggling."

Consider a story that illustrates the importance of intervention well: "Love you hon, see you soon." These were the last words spoken over the phone by widower Paul Dispenza to his wife Melissa on January 28, 2013. Moments later, Melissa was being rushed by ambulance to the Erie County Medical Center, mortally injured when struck by a car. Melissa was 54 years old and a mother of two. "I was numb," said Paul. "I didn't sleep for three days. The low point was a day later, when I pounded my head against the cellar wall, not wanting to live anymore without Melissa. I sobbed uncontrollably. I knew I was in trouble and had better reach for help. I called a friend of the family named Katie, who came over within five minutes. She held me for some time as I cried harder than any baby is able to cry." Paul said it was Katie who helped him realize he needed medical attention. "I went to see my doctor, who prescribed an antidepressant."

Suicide

Research has shown that widowers are at a greater risk of suicide than widows. A Swiss study of people whose spouses died found that about one in every 2,300 widows committed suicide in the first year, while the rate for widowers was almost four times higher—one in every 600. And men are already more likely to commit suicide. Men account for 79% of deaths by suicide in the U.S. If I don't have your attention already, let me put an even finer point on it: Suicide among widowers is most likely during *the first week* after the death of their spouse. And suicide rates remain high for about three years. Socioeconomic status doesn't play a role. Rich or poor, widowers are at risk.

Eric Brown, who lost his partner Carleton Cannon in 2013, credits a friend who needed a place to stay for four months with saving his life. That was a fortunate coincidence, because, as Eric says, "I wasn't able to get on the phone to ask for help because of my grief." Other than Eric's close friends, few others even visited him or checked to see if he was okay following his loss. He suggests that this may occur because, "In our society, many people are uncomfortable with death." Eric adds that when you are widowed, "All of your strengths disappear. Grieving supersedes other skills and feelings."

Widower Steve Marquardt lost his appetite and had difficulty sleeping. "I did have thoughts of suicide so that I could be with

Merethe. There were times when I would be driving to work on the freeway and think, *I could just drive off the road right here and end everything.* But then I thought of the kids and came to my senses. I decided to see my doctor for my depression, and he prescribed some medications. I surrounded myself with good friends who helped me a lot."

A widower who recognizes suicidal thoughts should "surround himself with supportive people, and if in a state of crisis call a suicide prevention hotline," Zimmer says. He adds that "Family and friends should remove firearms [the rate of suicide rises dramatically if there's a gun in the house], if there are any, and encourage or even accompany the widower to see a therapist. They should stay connected and in touch with the widower without blaming or getting angry at him" for having suicidal thoughts.

Post-Traumatic Stress Disorder

Widowers sometimes suffer symptoms of post-traumatic stress disorder (PTSD), which can develop after someone is exposed to traumatic events. PTSD symptoms include recurring nightmares, panic attacks, hostility, and self-destructive behavior.

While PTSD is no longer thought to be exclusively associated with combat veterans, I did ask widower Chris Sweet, a U.S. Air Force Master Sergeant, whether or not he thought losing a spouse creates PTSD-like symptoms in widowers. "Absolutely," Chris said. As part of his duties, Chris held briefings to help military men and women reintegrate into society after returning from overseas, and those briefings included professionals who evaluated signs of PTSD.

Understanding the symptoms of PTSD as he does, Chris believes he experienced PTSD after the death of his wife, Jessica. His new wife, Danielle, whose husband was killed in Iraq, told us that "when Chris and I started dating, and then for a long time, he was in a very dark place. He drank quite a bit, so I think that's how he dealt with his grief." Chris added that PTSD should be a big topic when someone loses a spouse, but it isn't.

Research proves Chris right. A study by the University of California–San Diego of both widows and widowers found that two months after a spouse died from a chronic illness, 10% of surviving spouses suffered from PTSD. Also, 9% of those whose spouses died unexpectedly met the criteria for PTSD, and 36% of those whose spouses died from "unnatural" causes, meaning suicide or accident, had PTSD.

PTSD Symptoms

- Recurring nightmares
- Panic attacks
- Flashbacks: Acting or feeling as though the traumatic event were happening again
- Having extreme distress when reminded of the traumatic event
- A surge in your heart rate or sweating when recalling the event
- Blocking out memories
- Experiencing emotional blocks to positive emotions, such as happiness or love
- Thoughts of suicide
- Having a difficult time falling or staying asleep
- Increased rage or having outbursts of anger
- Difficulty concentrating
- Feeling constantly on guard or as if danger is everywhere
- Being jumpy or easily startled

Given these findings and Chris Sweet's observations and experiences, widowers need to play it safe by sharing any of these symptoms they are experiencing with their doctor.

Psychologist Zimmer says PTSD sufferers can go on undiagnosed, and their symptoms unresolved, for years. Then, upon the occurrence of yet another loss, the PTSD can resurface. The same can be said about unresolved grief. As an example, says Zimmer, "if the widower lost a sibling or parent as a child and never mourned that loss, it may exaggerate the emotional impact of the current loss, which could be confusing, scary and overwhelming." He recommends that the sufferer "consult with a psychologist, clinical social worker, or another specialist in talk therapy."

See a Doctor

As I said before, if you are like most men, your wife likely did more to monitor and improve your health then you ever did. With her passing, you need to take on this responsibility. To underscore: According to the U.S. Agency for Healthcare Research and Quality, men are 25% less likely to have visited a healthcare provider in the past year, and almost 40% more likely to have skipped recommended cholesterol screenings, placing their otherwise fragile health at even greater risk. Without exception, every widower should be seen by his doctor, but not at the exclusion of being seen by a psychotherapist.

Zimmer notes that some men are reluctant to see a grief counselor because they associate doing so with being weak or dependent. They say they don't believe in therapy, they don't need help, and they will handle their problems on their own. What's the expression? Pride goeth before a fall? If you need psychological help, get it. Therapy does not take independent, self-reliant men and make them helpless or dependent. It is not a sign of weakness; it's a sign you're smart enough to know you need some help. It will speed your journey to recovery, and if that isn't enough, it will make you psychologically stronger more quickly so you can better help your kids and others deal with the loss.

Says Zimmer: "As a man, I completely understand how we were socialized as young boys to be strong, and any display of emotion was often considered a weakness. When it comes to needing help from a financial advisor or a good mechanic, we don't hesitate. But when it comes to psychological help, feelings of shame can block us. A good therapist can help us fix that."

Following Michelle's death, I knew I needed to do what I could to ensure that my life was headed in the right direction. So I sought the counsel of both a Catholic priest and a counselor from a Veterans Administration hospital. Together, they were instrumental in keeping my feet moving forward on the path to recovery.

Employee Assistance Programs

Widowers who would like to visit with a mental health professional but may not have the right health insurance or resources to do so may want to see whether their employer has an employee assistance program (EAP). An EAP is one of the best benefits instituted by American employers, and it can help employees who are facing a family crisis.

EAPs often include free, confidential short-term counseling and referral services, available to both employees and members of their immediate family. Often a firm's EAP expert will refer the employee to an outside professional, where the employee will usually be able to receive a number of free services. Should additional services be needed, the employee would need to turn to their healthcare provider for coverage or find another way to cover the expense.

In the next chapter, we go into detail on another key benefit: The Family and Medical Leave Act.

EAP Benefits

EAPs can assist employees with a number of issues, including:

- Marriage
- Substance abuse
- Alcohol abuse
- Occupational stress
- Emotional distress or grief
- Major life events, including births, accidents, and deaths
- Healthcare concerns
- Financial or non-work-related legal concerns
- Family/personal relationship issues
- Work relationship issues
- Concerns about aging parents

Don't Take Chances

In spite of my efforts to stay healthy during the toughest period of my life, I was not only diagnosed with kidney stones within ten days of Michelle's passing, but I was also diagnosed with prostate cancer five years later. While I can't say for sure there was a correlation between these illnesses and the stress of serving as a caregiver for over three years, but it does raise questions.

According to a study comparing 200 kidney stone patients with 200 people without the condition, the patients were more likely to have had major stress in the past two years. The study, led by researcher Dr. G. Reza Najem, of the New Jersey Medical School at Rutgers University, described how stresses included the death of a loved one.

And while experts are still determining whether stress causes cancer, there is "little doubt that it promotes the growth and spread of some forms of the disease," says Markham Held, writing for the MD Anderson Cancer Center's website. MD Anderson's Dr. Lorenzo Cohen adds, "Stress makes your body more hospitable to cancer."

To summarize: While you may not ever have kidney disease, or be diagnosed with prostate cancer, if you have been a long-term caregiver, a widower, or both, you are vulnerable to falling prey to any number of ailments. Don't take chances. See your doctor regularly. Have your blood work done, including having your PSA (prostate-specific antigen) levels checked. Watch your weight and your blood pressure, and get exercise a few days each week, even if only for 15 minutes. Take your meds and vitamins. Avoid smoking, excessive use of alcohol, and drugs.

And ask your doctor if you should also see a mental health professional, or seek the help of one yourself if you think you need to.

CHAPTER 5

Help From a Higher Power

This chapter was written for those who seek to help their healing through spirituality. I'll share views and stories from our team of contributing widowers on the role their religious and spiritual beliefs had in their journeys, and how it eased their grief. Readers will also be introduced to our team of religious experts, including two Christian ministers, one Rabbi, and a Roman Catholic priest. Though I found comfort in my faith and will encourage widowers to renew and deepen their faith to help their recoveries, this is an honest look at religion. Some widowers will openly express their anger toward God and their reasons for discontinuing the practice of their faith.

Just as we said in Chapter 2 that there isn't one path to working through grief, there is no one path for healing through faith. As Rabbi Alexis Pearce tells us, "spirituality is a very delicate, personal and intimate thing." So if you're reading this book to help a widower you know, and you feel religion might do him some good, suggest it gingerly. Maybe invite him to play a round of golf in your church golf league, or ask him to help you with a church volunteer project.

The Bible speaks plainly on the help God gives those who grieve. Pastor Doug Fultz believes God is especially close to people who are heartbroken. He quoted Psalm 3:19 to me: "The Lord is close to the brokenhearted and saves those who are crushed in spirit," which comforted me. And the Bible calls upon the religious community to help those who have lost someone dear. "Blessed are those who mourn, for they shall be comforted" (Matthew 5:4). And we of faith are comforted that the Bible assures us that someday we will be re-united with our loved ones in heaven.

I cannot put into words the role of faith in healing our spiritual wounds better than Pastor Ken Hagin. Pastor Hagin says that at its most powerful, faith helps us establish a personal relationship with God. "It is within personal relationships that we experience loss, and consequently, it is within personal relationships where we find comfort and, more importantly, personal peace. God wants to be the provider of the peace that is being sought; so as we continue on our journey through the most difficult times in our lives, we need to re-member it is not in the inanimate rules of religion where one finds comfort but through a personal relationship with God."

I learned how widowers found many different ways for their faith to help them. Widower Bob Page, himself a minister, became ob-sessed with the word *alone* following the death of his wife, Linda. "I can't tell you how much that word penetrated my psyche. I was overwhelmed by the whole concept of it. John 16:32 describes how Jesus is headed toward the cross and says, 'Yet, I am not alone, for the Father is with me.' That verse became everything for me. It gave me comfort and perspective."

Widower Quentin Strode, a man of religious strength, says: "Through the tough times, based on my religious beliefs, I know I will see my beloved Shanda again. And knowing this has helped me to cope with my loss."

Sadly, grieving sometimes pushes some of us further away from our faith. Rabbi Pearce says bereaved people often tell her that during the anxious and exhausting days of caregiving and the miserable days of grief, they feel cut off from a connection to God. "They can't pray, they can't focus enough to meditate, and they don't feel like life is giving them any support."

And some feel anger at God, she says. She likes to tell people to be as angry at God as they want. God can take it. "You don't have to approve or agree with what is happening. In fact, fighting it is a sign of healthy defiance."

How Religion Helps

As a man of faith, I believe in the healing power of a personal relationship with God, as Pastor Hagin said. But I also recognize that religion is a balm unto itself. Rutgers University sociology professor Deborah Carr says that religion often helps the bereaved cope with their loss by providing two critical resources: social support and a worldview that helps them make sense of the death. "Congregations are filled with like-minded people who can provide emotional and practical help—everything from meals to rides to hands-on assistance when they are caring for their dying loved one. But religious communities also provide a set of beliefs that helps people make sense of their problems and come to peace with their lives."

Rabbi Pearce teaches us how "friendship and support may well come from a religious community. Particularly, if people have been involved in a small group, or synagogue *havurah*, they have a tight circle of close friends who do holidays and celebrations together and support each other in times of grief. Entering into a religious community can be beneficial if it's a place where the people and the message resonate and feel right. Many are drawn to the comforting rituals of their childhood, both as the end of life nears and as they grieve."

If the deceased was Jewish, a *shiva* might be performed. This is seven days of formal mourning just after a funeral of a close relative and is referred to as sitting shiva. There is another Jewish tradition that is important and may have special importance to a widower. *Minyan* is a group of 10 men, age 13 or older, who are needed to recite the Kaddish prayer, or prayer for the dead, at funerals and home shiva. Having men attend to the spiritual needs of a fellow man gives special support often lacking for widowers, given that men often find it hard to comfort a fellow man.

Those who practice other faiths may discover grief support groups that serve the same purpose: people to share with, and who understand and welcome you.

Catherine Sanderson, a psychology professor at Amherst College, has studied things that we *think* will make us happy but don't, as well as things that really do make us happy. In a *Washington Post* story, she was quoted as saying a study found that "the secret to sustained happiness lies in participation in religion. Researchers looked at four areas: volunteering or working with a charity; taking educational courses; participating in religious organizations, and participating in a political or community organization. Of the four, participating in a religious organization was the only social activity associated with sustained happiness."

And this study was skewed toward older people, who are much more likely to be widows or widowers: It surveyed 9,000 Europeans who were over the age of 50. Mauricio Avendano, an epidemiologist and an author of the study, wrote, "The church appears to play a very important social role in keeping depression at bay and also as a coping mechanism during periods of illness in later life."

Pastor Fultz teaches us that happiness can often be dependent on what happens to you. But *joy* is a deeper sense of peace and hope that is there no matter what happens to you. Joy is one of the fruits of the Holy Spirit, he says.

Widower Phil Carbone says his faith provided him with greater strength and wisdom when dealing with the aftermath of his wife Lisa's passing, adding, "Although you wouldn't have been able to validate my view with my church attendance record." Widower Norris Jergenson says his religion not only helped him during the events surrounding the death of his wife, Darlene, but it continues to do so to this day.

"Without my faith in God, I would not have been able to deal with my loss," says double widower Earnest Moran. "He says He will not let us go through more than His grace will sustain us. I know my wife went to be with her Lord when she died, and the Bible says I will see her again." Earnest's brother, widower Harold Moran (who you may recall is also a double widower), says, "So far, my faith is the only thing I have to lean on. Knowing that God has a plan for me keeps me going."

> *When anxiety was great within me, your consolation brought me joy.*
>
> *Psalm 94:19*

Anger at God

Anger at God is a common reaction of widowers, even those of deep faith. But the result of that anger can be very different among them. A devoted Catholic and a deacon in the Catholic Church (later to be ordained a Catholic priest), widower Gregg Elliott said he felt "great anger" when he lost his beloved Janette. "I felt Janette had been cheated out of life. And even though I was a deacon in the Catholic Church, I felt God had let her down. By the pain she suffered and her death, she was cheated of the reward of a long and fruitful retirement, to see her kids grow up and have children and enjoy life as a grandparent. I guess even clergy are not immune to the pain a widower experiences. I carried that anger nearly a year."

Father Elliott went on: "About one year following Janette's death, and with Easter approaching, I read *The Passion of Christ*. I saw how much Christ suffered, how scared he was, and the fear of the pain he faced. And yet, he was able to say, 'I'll do it.' God's son suffered because of his love for us. I came to realize that if Jesus suffered as I did so that my sins could be forgiven, I knew he was there for both Janette and me. After that realization, I was able to move on, and I was able then to make a decision to leave Houston, where I was living, and get my life started as a hospital chaplain in Oklahoma.

"Admittedly, it took the help of a psychologist over a period to help me to take a look at all of the other things that were going on. That helped me to see a path. When I did, I gave up a close relationship that had started after Jeannette died with someone who had lost her spouse. I made a decision to see what else God had in store for me. I know that was the right decision to make as my new life unfolded, presenting me with an open door to becoming a priest."

Some widowers with whom we spoke described how they lost faith in religion or turned their back on their religious teachings as they watched their wives suffer. Rabbi Pearce points out how it is common to interpret pain as punishment and to feel God is punishing you when a loved one is taken. "This can lead to guilt when people look for the wrong they must have done to result in this punishment," says Pearce. "And it can lead to anger if the death is perceived as wrongful." Pearce continues, "Still, many people question the meaning of life and the reality of God when grief is fresh." For example, widower John Von Der Haar has deep-rooted anger about God. "I grew up Catholic, and later drifted away from religion altogether. Mary's passing has created bitterness and anger I have never felt before. If anything, Mary's passing has made me less religious. I am still angry at God for taking Mary away too early. What kind of benevolent being would create something like cancer? I am not religious anymore, and I cannot imagine there is anything beyond this life."

John isn't alone in his feelings of anger toward God. Following the loss of his wife Dawn, widower Tony Cabuno said, "I had to blame someone, so I guess it had to be God." Tony sent his son Dante to religious instruction classes at his church. "While I was there, I asked a priest to speak with me. I yelled at him for 20 minutes. Yeah, I was mad at God."

For others, the anger is short-lived, and after a break, these widowers return to their religious communities. Widower and U.S. Air Force Master Sergeant Chris Sweet stayed away from his church for the first year following the death of his wife, Jessica. "I felt too much anger." Both Chris and his current wife Danielle lost a spouse who was serving in the military. Danielle revealed how she and her then-husband Ryan attended church regularly, but after he was killed in action while serving in Iraq, Danielle said, "I honestly did not want anything to do with God because I did not understand how he could allow us to lose Ryan."

Rabbi Pearce explains how Jewish beliefs teach how the mourner is encouraged to see their loss as part of God's overall design, not a personal attack. Pearce adds, "We are asked to admit that we never owned our loved one; they came from mystery, they go to mystery." This is provided for in scripture.

From dust we came, and to dust we return.
Genesis 3:19

Finding Your Own Path

Not all widowers have a need for a religious community and instead find their own spiritual path. Widower Rob Hagen met with a group of six or seven friends each month, during which time they explored questions around spirituality. "We weren't looking to embrace any dogma, any structure. In fact, we tried to avoid the church. For me, there has been a newfound curiosity about going back and revisiting my old ideas around spirituality to see what resonates, what makes sense to me now. For a long time, so much did not make sense to me,

I rejected it all." He says that the passing of his partner, Larry, "has indirectly and suddenly triggered a new spiritual quest or questioning in me that has been pretty good, pretty cool."

> *My soul is weary with sorrow; strengthen me according to your word.*
>
> *Psalm 119:28*

> *The Lord is my strength and my shield; my heart trusts in him, and he helps me. My heart leaps for joy, and with my song I praise him.*
>
> *Psalm 28:7*

I believe all houses of worship serve the same basic purpose. That said, widowers may find they are more comfortable in one environment versus another. There is nothing wrong with visiting other churches, temples, synagogues, mosques, or religious centers and experiencing their teachings and programs. Widower Ralph McNiven visited a Methodist Church, to sort of comparison shop. He discovered he was more comfortable with the Episcopal Church.

The Power of Prayer

In Luke 11:1, Jesus' disciples asked, "Lord, teach us to pray." Sadly, many people have never been taught how to pray, causing them to avoid doing so, even when they wish they could. There many resources available that can assist you in learning how to pray if you have difficulty getting started. Of course, a religious leader can help you, but you may want to explore different ways to pray and create your own method. Google it—there's a long list of resources available.

Whether one is Protestant, Catholic, Jewish, Muslim, or another faith, prayer has its place in our daily lives. And we often turn to the power of prayer, especially to help others. A Baylor University study found that 90% of Americans have prayed for healing, for example. Pastor Fultz reminds us of how David, the author of most Psalms, relied on prayer. Psalm 116.l: "I love the Lord, for he heard my voice; he heard my cry for mercy. Because he turned his ear to me, I will call on him as long as I live."

I believe there is something to be said for *unanswered prayers*. Those who pray sometimes ask for things in prayer that are not in their best interest. Sometimes, by not fulfilling a prayer request, God answered your prayer.

This power of unanswered prayers was well put in a song co-written and recorded by country star Garth Brooks. Titled *Unanswered Prayers*, the song's lyrics describe a man who was attending a hometown football game with his wife when he ran into an old girlfriend. He recalled when he dated the former girlfriend that he would offer a silent prayer, asking God to "make her mine." As his life would play out, God had different plans for him, and he married someone else. Much like the message contained in that Garth Brooks song, I believe unanswered prayers are, in fact, God's answers. The faithful need to keep their mind and eyes receptive to receive God's messages, even those that come in the form of unanswered prayers, for they too are gifts from the Almighty.

Pastor Fultz shares with us the story of a couple who came to a church service asking for healing after the woman had been diagnosed with cancer. The evangelist prayed for them and anointed them with oil. Months later, the evangelist received a call from the husband, thanking him for praying for his wife, saying it was the most powerful and healing experience they had ever had. The evangelist thought the wife was healed and the cancer was gone. But when he asked how she was doing, the husband said she had died just a few days earlier. The evangelist was shaken. He was certain that God had healed the woman, and said, "I'm so sorry about your loss." The widower said, "Don't be sorry. Before we came to that church service, my wife was very bitter about God. She believed God had forgotten her. Her bitterness spread to the rest of the family, and she never smiled and was always critical and negative. But after your prayer for her, everything changed. There was a peace that came over her. During the last few months of her life, we laughed, sang, and had more meaningful talks than we had during all the rest of our marriage." And then he said, "God decided not to cure my wife of cancer. But he healed her."

The Lord is trustworthy in all he promises and faithful in all he does. The Lord upholds all who fall and lifts up all who are bowed down.

Psalm 145:13,14

Before moving to the Nashville area in 2002, I wasn't that familiar with the practice of making prayer lists. Following Michelle's diagnosis, several people, including many of my colleagues at Bank of America, approached me and mentioned how they had added Michelle's name to their church's prayer list. I have come to believe in the power of prayer. I have seen it work. Most recently, I witnessed its powers at Lourdes in France, where stricken individuals from around the world travel to drink and bathe in the waters. The number of abandoned wheelchairs, crutches, and verbal testimonies attest to the miraculous healings that take place there.

I'll close this section about prayer with this poem, attributed to a Confederate soldier near the end of the Civil War, and which reflects my views pretty well.

A Confederate Soldier's Prayer

Author Unknown
(attributed to a battle-weary C.S.A. soldier near the end of the war)

I asked God for strength, that I might achieve
I was made weak, that I might learn humbly to obey.

I asked for health, that I might do great things,
I was given infirmity, that I might do better things.

I asked for riches, that I might be happy,
I was given poverty, that I might be wise.

I asked for power, that I might have the praise of men,
I was given weakness, that I might feel the need of God

I asked for all things, that I might enjoy life,
I was given life, that I might enjoy all things.

I got nothing that I asked for, but everything I had hoped for.
Almost despite myself, my unspoken prayers were answered.

I am, among all men, most richly blessed.

Religion and My Story

In this final section, I'll talk about how my religious beliefs served me during my time of need.

Raised a Catholic, I attended a Catholic grade school where Felician sisters were the teachers. Admittedly, I wasn't the best

Catholic in my younger days, but I always believed in God, and deep down inside I saw myself as Catholic. My faith has been a quiet constant in my life.

Michelle was raised a Methodist. So that our family would be able to worship together, I attended a Methodist Church during the eight years we lived near Albany, N.Y. Later, we moved to Nashville, and still later to San Antonio, where we worshiped at non-denominational Christian churches. Regardless of where we found ourselves praying, I didn't need to be in a Catholic church to practice my faith. No matter where I worshiped, I knew God knew who I was, knew everything that was going on in my life, and was concerned about the issues in my life.

As many of you know, when your wife is diagnosed with a serious illness, a sense of helpless falls upon you. You begin grasping at anything that may, even in a small way, comfort your ailing spouse, or provide a distraction from your fears. Where does one turn? I turned toward God.

There is no doubt in my mind that He was with me during the tough days that I served as a caregiver for Michelle, as well as during the long and dark days that followed Michelle's passing. And I frankly could not have made it without my church and those who ministered to me. Without exception, each day I felt God's presence. I knew my savior was guiding my thoughts, and my efforts to provide for my stricken wife with the best medical care possible. Time and time again, I knew I was being influenced and supported by the gentle hands of Jesus, as was Michelle.

Cast all our anxiety on him because he cares for you.
1 Peter 5:7

No matter how ill Michelle became, and no matter how close she came to death, she would frequently say, "God will have his way." So strong was her faith, Michelle was able to draw comfort in knowing

God was at her side. And this support enabled her to live as normal a life as possible during her battle with cancer.

The thirty-nine months of Michelle's illness were the best of times during our sixteen years of marriage. Our faith in our Lord had much to do with the peace that came upon us. Like the widower Pastor Fultz speaks about, I, too, am at peace with the loss of Michelle. I do not feel cheated in any way. As my brother David said, Michelle and I had sixteen years of heaven when many couples have none. During Michelle's illness, she was able to teach me how I needed to do more for those less fortunate. When the average pancreatic cancer patient prognosis is usually measured in months if not weeks, Michelle's was measured in years—years during which she continuously touched the lives of others. And I got to watch one of God's greatest works in action.

In Chapter 1, I told you a little bit about how I came to recognize the existence of God's angels swirling around Michelle with the purpose of attending to her ever need. How a young angel doctor discovered Michelle's cancer when others did not, and that her radiology results showed she was eligible for a special surgical procedure that could save her life, which most pancreatic cancer patients are not. And how our angel neighbors ran to her side to comfort her, and that her case was accepted by another angel who happen to be one of the top surgeons in the world. How God provided Michelle with a wonderful distraction when a litter of nine beautiful golden retriever puppies was born to love just twenty-four hours after Michelle's diagnosis. Yes, Michelle had angels all around her. Michelle's Angels, to be exact.

I'd like to tell you about a profound moment of faith I experienced, and how it changed me. At about 11 p.m. on a stormy January evening in 2005, I was awaiting the arrival of my life-long friend, Edward Zimmer, who would be with me during Michelle's risky surgery. I felt a need to pray. Suddenly, I experienced a near supernatural exchange with God. I begged God to spare Michelle's life.

As I looked out over the parking ramp's fourth-story wall, my hands grasped in prayer; I suddenly felt a sustained and fierce wind racing past me, with lightning cracking in the sky above. I felt the Lord was with Michelle and me, and that he heard my fervent prayer. That moment in Houston was the closest I have ever felt to my God. The moment lives with me still and gives me comfort.

> *"Lord, you alone are my portion and my cup; you make my lot secure. The boundary lines have fallen for me in pleasant places; surely I have a delightful inheritance."*
>
> *Psalm 16:5, 6*

But there were other episodes that affected us both. Five months after Michelle's surgery, and following two close calls with death, Michelle was declared cancer-free in June 2005. Hallelujah! But in October 2005, Michelle and I traveled once again to Houston's MD Anderson Cancer Center for a follow-up visit, and we learned that Michelle's cancer had returned. Stunned, we returned to Houston's Hobby Airport for our return flight to Nashville.

As Michelle sat in our gate's waiting area, I stepped away to get something to drink. When I returned, I found Michelle speaking with a woman who had missed her flight to Minnesota. When Michelle and I were once again alone, I asked, "What was that about?" Michelle said the woman had walked up to her and asked, "Do you have cancer?" Michelle replied, "Yes, just two hours ago, I learned that my cancer had returned." Then the woman said, "I thought so. You have that *look*." The woman then added, "I have cancer, too. So you are the reason God had me miss my flight to Minnesota. He wanted us to meet."

God does work in mysterious ways. And if we're not careful, we'll miss His messages. Michelle and the angel from Minnesota communicated privately for months following their meeting. I am certain their relationship comforted Michelle during her long battle with cancer. I never learned her identity, but I pray Michelle's Minnesota Angel knows how much Michelle appreciated their friendship and how much I appreciated her willingness to sacrifice in the service of others.

Shortly after Michelle's death, I received an excited call from Michelle's good friend Ariane Montemuro, who lived across the street from us when we lived in Tennessee. The day before, Ariane said, she was thinking about Michelle while out for a walk. She made a prayer, asking Michelle to provide a sign to show Michelle was okay and in the presence of Our Lord. "Anything, just send me a sign."

Later that night, heavy rains and winds hit the Nashville area, causing some tree limbs to fall off nearby trees. When Ariane examined the debris the next morning, she looked across the street to the house where Michelle and I use to live. As she looked up, she saw how three tree limbs had fallen onto the roof of our old home, forming the letter "A." Ariane and I believe it was Michelle's response to Ariane's prayer, and that the letter "A" stood for Ariane or the word *angel*. Ariane was one of the original Michelle's Angels.

When Michelle and I lived in Nashville, we attended the Franklin Christian Church, a non-denominational house of worship where we were very comfortable. Shortly before Michelle passed away, she shared with me how she was baptized at the Franklin Community Church without any fanfare or notice provided to me.

Following Michelle's death, I subconsciously searched for ways to be closer to her. Even though we were living in San Antonio at the time of her death, when it came time to plan for Michelle's memorial service, I decided to hold it in Nashville at the Franklin Community Church. This was the house of worship Michelle loved the best.

As I planned Michelle's memorial service, I asked Pastor Fultz to baptize me in the same waters Michelle was baptized in a few months earlier. He did so the day before Michelle's memorial service was held. Although I was baptized as a child in the Catholic Church, I'm sure God didn't mind that I wanted to be baptized a second time.

Shortly after Michelle's passing, I felt a need to return to my religious roots. I called the pastor of my nearby Catholic Church in San Antonio and made an appointment to meet with him. Still grieving over the loss of Michelle, I opened my heart to my God during what became a tearful meeting, and I rejoined the Catholic Church. The priest heard my confession and then blessed me while placing his hands on my head. I must tell you, at that very moment, I felt an energy race through me. I like to think it was the Holy Spirit empowering me to write this book. I felt I had returned home. There is something comforting about revisiting the teachings that were originally introduced to us by our parents that is very much akin to a safe haven. I remember how I was moved by the realization of how much I missed the church of my youth.

"Come unto me all you who are weary and heavy laden— and I will give you rest."

Matthew 11:28

Some people have said to me in recent years how they did not realize I was so religious. My reply has been that I have always had a strong faith; I just didn't feel a need to share it until now. Today, I find I am more willing to express my faith openly. I have also discovered that I have adopted a new willingness to minister to others who may be hurting and are in need of comfort, regardless of the faith or religion they may practice if any. I'm certain that being exposed for five years to the culture in Nashville—a community some say is the belt buckle of the Bible Belt—helped give me the courage to express my faith more openly.

I know that some readers do not have a relationship with God. But hopefully in this chapter I've shown that such a relationship and the community provided by one's religion can be powerful sources of comfort and healing.

CHAPTER 6

Managing Your Career

"Time and tide wait for no man," wrote 14th-century poet Geoffrey Chaucer, and neither does a career. This chapter will talk about strategies to maintain your career as best you can during your wife's illness and following her passing; it will review your rights, and it will show how work can be a vital part of your recovery.

In some cases, when serving as a caregiver, losing ground in your career is inevitable. I'm an example of that. During my caregiver days, I did what I could to fulfill my professional duties. But given that Michelle was my priority, I wasn't working for my employer the way I (or they) wished I could have. At Farm Bureau Bank I led the retail side of the business, which included marketing, product management, and consumer, commercial, small business, and home lending. Within three months of arriving in Texas, Michelle's health began to deteriorate rapidly. Over the final ten weeks of her life, I was at her side and away from my office most of the time. During those weeks, the CEO restructured the bank and hired another executive to take over the lending functions that had been mine to lead. If I'd been the CEO, I would have done the same thing. Losing those responsibilities was collateral damage in the war to save Michelle's life. But later I realized I got off easy, and I'm grateful to this day to Farm Bureau Bank CEO Larry Lanie for the flexibility he gave me when caring for Michelle, and for not cutting my pay.

Widower Phil Carbone faced similar problems. He and his wife, Lisa, moved to the Baltimore area in 2001, two years after Lisa was first diagnosed with cancer. She was 49 when she died. Carbone said, "While my employer was supportive during our ordeal, the amount of time I needed to care for Lisa did hurt my career. Opportunities for promotions coincided with the time I was a caregiver. Unfortunately, I missed those promotions, and I have never been able to gain back that ground professionally." Still, Phil says, "I have no regrets; I made the right choice and would do it again."

What to Expect

When we're struggling with a loved one's death, seeing beyond our own situation is hard. We might think that our employers owe us, given the ordeal we've been through. But the world doesn't work that way, and employers have a job to do, no matter how grief-stricken their employees are. And no matter how valuable you think you are to your employer, don't expect special consideration.

Depending on your family situation, you may want to request a voluntary demotion to a less stressful position until after the most difficult of periods of caregiving and mourning have passed. Perhaps a role that will let you avoid corporate travel and give you more time to care for your children. I have seen some firms that will not only accommodate a loyal employee but also preserve his current salary when doing so. The employer certainly has the option to freeze an employee's salary at current levels during the time he may be away from his duties or serve in a lesser position. Once you're back on your feet, you should let your employer know that you're available for a more demanding role.

And an employer may be willing to provide all kinds of extra help, from free daycare to flexible employment hours.

At some point—perhaps before you're ready—you will be expected to return to work. In many ways, returning to work can be therapeutic. Work provides structure to the day and a sense of purpose. Most people function better when they have a purpose or goals they can contribute to, as discussed in Chapter 3. Besides, a break from the grieving can't hurt. Our careers, responsibilities, and duties provide the purpose that reassures us of our value to others.

Some of us rush back to work because it may be the only environment in which we feel comfortable or because we want to take our minds off of our grief. Perhaps this is why I chose to start my workday at before 5 a.m. and then keep going until my energy was spent. Besides, I wasn't eager to enter my empty home and confront the memories that waited for me there.

But work is more than just the bundle of tasks we do in a day. It also provides us social support and community. Widower Ralph MacNiven, an insurance agent from Ft. Myers, Florida, won a Mediterranean cruise from his company but didn't intend to go. When I asked why, he told me how he could function well at work, but not in social settings. "People didn't know what to say to me, and I didn't know what to say to them," Ralph said. As a result, he didn't want to be captive in a social environment for an entire week with colleagues and friends, and he feared he might be the object of pity. As things turned out, a close friend persuaded him to go at the last minute. Ralph later told me how beneficial the trip was and how grateful he was that his friend cared enough to offer the encouragement.

Widower Rutilo Flores had a similar experience. "I needed to keep myself busy following Raka's death, so I went out and got multiple part-time jobs. Money wasn't an issue for me; I just didn't want to come home or be alone. I needed to keep my mind and body busy thinking about something else. Even to this day, five years after my loss, I still hold multiple jobs."

Professor Carr tells us work means different things to widowers. "Some cope with their sadness by filling their hours with activity," like Rutilo. "Time and energy spent focusing on tasks are times not spent ruminating over one's loss, or hours spent stewing in one's own thoughts at home. But for others, keeping busy may not be effective. Those who attempt to hide in work while neglecting their feelings of loss and sorrow may find that those feelings return powerfully later. Know thyself. If you need time for peace and quiet, take it. If you prefer to channel your grief into a project or activity, then do so."

Widower Carl Jahrstorfer also focused single-mindedly on his work in his early years as a widower, but then recognized that there was a better path for him. As Carl explained, "For the first three years following Pat's passing, my work kept me busy. But then, suddenly, the loneliness factor multiplied by tenfold." That's when Carl recognized that he needed to address his issues head-on.

There is much to consider when determining the best time to return to work. While each of us ultimately makes this decision on our own, I recommend making it after visiting with your doctor, a mental health professional, and perhaps a trusted member of your Personal Advisory Board (see Chapter 2). In hindsight, I know I wish I had.

You may find one of your co-workers volunteering to be a sounding board or to help you and your family in different ways. One colleague may volunteer to perform some of your duties while you are away, while another may voluntarily offer to speak on your behalf with management as they make provisions for your particular needs. The key word here is *volunteer*. You should not *expect* such support, given that your co-workers are not obliged to help.

According to Robert Zucker, the founder and director of Caring Communities Respond, a New England consortium that offers bereavement counseling, "supervisors and co-workers form an important support system. Employees who experience a compassionate response to their situation often become intensely loyal." And he adds that co-workers who see supervisors going above and beyond to help an employee also feel more loyal to their employer.

Dr. Carr points out that most relationships in this world are reciprocal. A co-worker may help us today, but we are likely to pay it back by helping him when he encounters his own struggles in the future. When we take a long-term look at our workplace relationships, we may well remember many such examples of helping.

Re-Evaluating Work

Following the loss of a spouse, some men will reevaluate their careers, or perhaps even revisit their own commitment to their company. Some will elect to move on to another firm; some will change careers entirely. Some may feel that change will soften the grief they are experiencing. If you are a widower considering major a career move, move slowly. I've spoken to enough widowers to know many who regretted making hasty decisions while under duress.

To help take the emotion out of such a decision, consider some hard questions about a potential new employer:

- Is the new employer's work environment truly better, or are you imaging it is because you want a change?
- Are you giving up pension benefits by leaving your current employer?
- Can you work long enough at the new employer to become vested in their pension plan?
- How do the benefits compare?
- Would staying with your current employer offer more or less job security?

If there's one thing that widowers and professionals alike agree on, it's that you must not make a major decision when you're feeling highly emotional. Write down the pluses and minuses of change, and then revisit the list regularly for a week or even a month or two. At some point, your logical brain will kick into gear, and that may change your thinking entirely. You don't want to look back after making a hasty decision and discover that your impulsive actions just cost you a sizable bonus, stock options, a promotion, or some other benefit that your new employer is unable to match.

However, the way your employer treats employees may give you some justification for moving on. I worked at such a company. The company decided to lay off a small number of employees, and in the process of doing so, it let go an employee who had been diagnosed with cancer. To me, the management lacked the compassion I would want to see provided to one in need. Such an employer doesn't deserve the loyalty of its employees.

Looking Forward

I want to end this chapter with a story about how important work relationships can be to recovery, and how I received a gift from a co-worker during one of my darkest days. That co-worker was Enrique Lerma, and he was the head of the collections department at Farm Bureau Bank. But I'll let Enrique tell the story, as he related it to my editor, Bob Frick:

"I liked Herb from the beginning. He had a great attitude and this wonderful, deep voice, which reminded me of Paul Harvey's. Every time Herb talked about Michelle, his face would light up. He was madly in love with her. She was the air that he breathed. She was already sick when I met him, and I think Herb did his best to remain positive. Toward the end, when he knew there wasn't much time left, I could tell he was getting a little sadder with each day. He's typically a high-spirited guy, and up to that point, he was still very positive.

Toward the end, I could tell it was tearing him up inside. But he didn't want Michelle to know.

"When she died, the difference was like night and day. I wasn't close to him, but when he came back he was very distant, and I was careful not to approach him too soon after her death. But I could tell many of his fellow executives at the bank didn't seem to care about how he was doing, and I didn't see them even trying to take him to lunch. Ninety percent of the time, the door of Herb's office was closed. But sometimes I could hear sad songs coming from his office, like the Carpenters.

"I was hoping his peers would step in, but they didn't. For weeks on end he didn't come out of his office. Finally, I took a chance, and I decided to knock on his door one day after work. I said, 'You know what, Herb? Log off your computer. I'm taking you to dinner.' Reluctantly, he agreed, and what I thought would be a two-hour dinner turned into three or four. Two bottles of wine turned into three, and then four, and then two desserts.

"We didn't necessarily talk about Michelle. He talked about how he was so concerned about being a good father to his stepson. And I remember him saying, 'I'm hurting really badly, Enrique, but if I had to do it all over again, I would.' "

It took courage, not to mention compassion, for Enrique to approach me as he did. By reaching out to me that summer evening, he helped me complete one of the critical steps of my healing and helped me out of the depths of my grief. For this, I can never repay him.

Contributing Widowers

I admire the men on the following pages for their generosity and bravery in helping with this book. I include this section because I thought readers would want to learn a little more about their lives and have a look at the men who lent their stories to help fellow widowers. If you would like to contact one or more of the this book's contributing widowers you can write to Widower's Support Network, 1730 Dogwood Forest Way, Lake Mary, Florida 32746 or write us at herb@WidowersSupportNetwork.com.

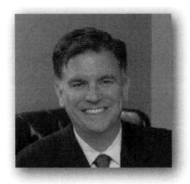

Contributing Widower: Eric Brown
Career: Financial Advisor
Residence: San Diego, California
Lost his partner Carleton Cannon (29) on 8/20/13
Cause of Death: Cancer/AIDS

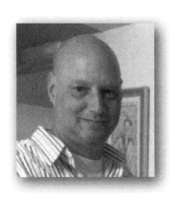

Contributing Widower: Tony Cabuno
Career: Sales Management
Residence: Struthers, Ohio
Lost his wife Dawn Cabuno (40) on 9/8/07
Cause of Death: Breast Cancer

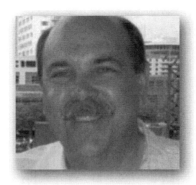

Contributing Widower: Philip Carbone
Career: Banking Executive
Residence: Amherst, New York
Lost his wife Lisa Saviola Carbone (49) on 11/15/2005.
Cause of Death: Metastatic Breast Cancer.

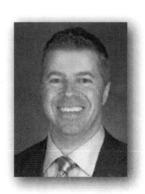

Contributing Widower & Subject Matter Expert: Mark Colgan
Career: Financial Planner
Residence: Honeoye Falls, New York
Lost his wife Joanne Colgan (28) on 9/4/01
Cause of Death: Congenital heart disease

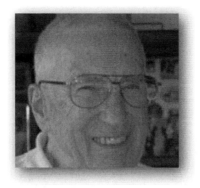

Contributing Widower: Doug Covert
Career: College Professor
Residence: St. Augustine, Florida
Lost his wife Caroline Dow (62) on 9/4/2004.
Cause of Death: Pancreatic Cancer.

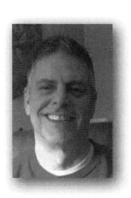

Contributing Widower: Paul Dispenza
Career: Bartender
Residence: Eggertsville, New York
Lost his wife Melissa Dispenza (54) on 1/28/13
Cause of Death: Struck by car

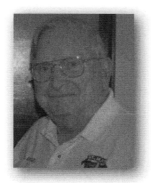

Contributing Widower and Subject Matter Expert: Rev. Gregg Elliott, LTC USAF (ret.)
Career: U.S. Air Force – Catholic Priest
Residence: Clinton, Washington
Lost his wife Janette Irene (55) on 3/25/96
Cause of Death: Cancer

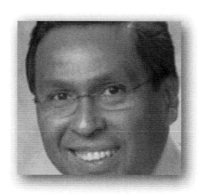

Contributing Widower: Rutilo Flores
Career: Naval Architectural Engineer
Residence: Chicago, Illinois
Lost his wife Raka Kumari (57) on 6/13/11
Cause of Death: Breast Cancer

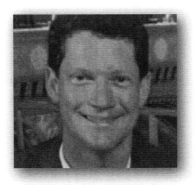

Contributing Widower: Jeff Gower
Career: Financial Advisor
Residence: Summerfield, Florida
Lost his wife Susan Gower (48) on 4/19/05
Cause of Death: Ovarian Cancer

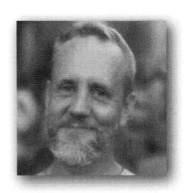

Contributing Widower: Rod Hagan
Career: Project Manager
Residence: Palm Springs, California
Lost his partner Larry Lambert (65) on 9-12-2011
Cause of Death: Cancer

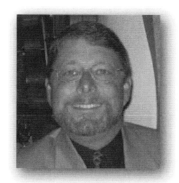

Contributing Widower: John Heffernan
Career: Sales
Residence: Orlando, Florida
Lost his wife Mary Heffernan (56) on 5/8/13
Cause of Death: Lung Cancer

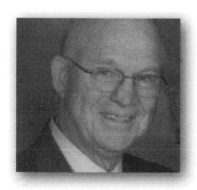

Contributing Widower: Carl Jahrstorfer
Career: Director of Development in the Senior Housing Industry
Residence: Wilmington, North Carolina
Lost his wife Patricia Jahrstorfer (68) on 4/6/12
Cause of Death: Ovarian Cancer

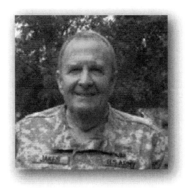

Contributing Widower: Col. Brian P. Jakes (ret)
Career: CEO: Health Education Organization
Residence: Mandeville, Louisiana
Lost his wife Luci Jakes (46) on 2/23/89
Cause of Death: Metastatic Breast Cancer

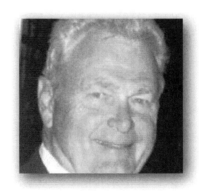

Contributing Widower: Norris Jergenson
Career: Director of Materials
Residence: The Villages, Florida
Lost his wife Darlene Jergenson (69) on 7/4/12
Cause of Death: Ovarian Cancer

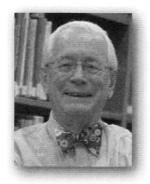

Contributing Widower: Nyle Kardatzke
Career: Private school headmaster
Residence: Indianapolis, Indiana
Lost his wife Darlene Sayers Kardatzke (64) on 10/25/10
Cause of Death: Metastatic breast cancer

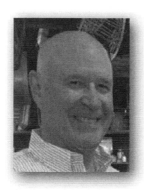

Contributing Widower: Ralph MacNiven
Career: Insurance Agent
Residence: Naples, Florida
Lost his wife Donna MacNiven (63) on 11/30/11
Cause of Death: Breast Cancer

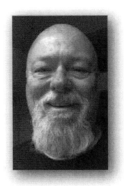

Contributing Widower: Steve Marquardt
Career: Auto Technician for the LAPD
Residence: Rancho Cucamonga, California
Lost his wife Merethe Marquardt (40) on 11/27/1996
Cause of Death: Acute NonLymphoblastic Leukemia

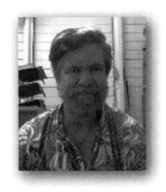

Contributing Widower: Keith Merriam
Career: Educator/Bookstore Manager
Residence: Kaneohe, Hawaii
Lost his wife Suzy Williams Merriam (44) on 9-19-99
Cause of Death: Breast Cancer

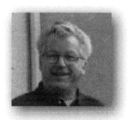

Contributing Widower: Earnest Moran
Career: Power Plant Mechanic/Machinist
Residence: Yuma, Arizona
Lost his first wife Dianna Marie Moran (67) 2/7/2009
Cause of Death: Auto accident

Lost his second wife Marge Moran (78) 11/11/2010
Cause of Death: Pancreatic Cancer

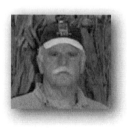

Contributing Widower: Harold Moran
Career: Senior Field Engineer
Residence: Johnston, New York
Lost his first wife Constance L. Moran (48) 10/19/2006
Cause of Death: Breast Cancer

Lost his second wife Barbara J. Moran (55) on 4/21/2013
Cause of Death: Brain Hemorrhage

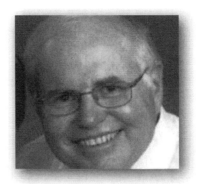

Contributing Widower: Pastor Robert (Bob) Page
Career: Church Pastor
Residence: The Village, Florida
Lost his wife Linda Page (60) on 2/27/09
Cause of Death: Kidney cancer

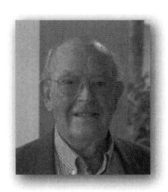

Contributing Widower: Bruce (Bud) Savage
Career: Sales, Utility and Cement industries
Residence: The Villages, Florida
Lost his wife Margaret Savage (80) on 8-13-11
Cause of Death: Heart Failure

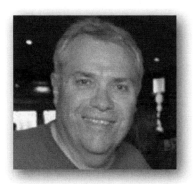

Contributing Widower: Robert Schlieper
Career: Banking Systems Information Technology
Residence: The Villages, Florida
Lost his wife Marian Schlieper (50) 12/28/2004
Cause of Death: Lung Cancer

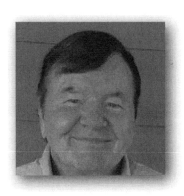

Contributing Widower: Gary Secor
Career: Software Project Manager
Residence: Suwanee, Georgia
Lost his wife Susan Jo Reich (64) on 12/14/12
Cause of Death: Long illness

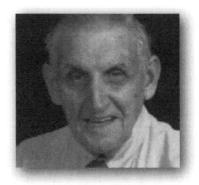

Contributing Widower: Aaron Seiden
Career: Federal Civil Service Employee
Residence: Baltimore, Maryland
Lost his wife Lorraine Seiden (56) on 1/23/86
Cause of Death: Heart Failure

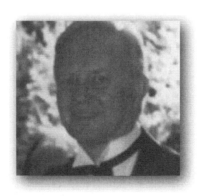

Contributing Widower: Otto Souder
Career: Bank Executive
Residence: The Villages, Florida
Lost his wife Dolly Garvin Souder (83) on 9/17/10
Cause of Death: Undisclosed

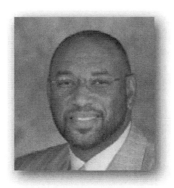

Contributing Widower: Quentin Strode
Career: Bank and Business Executive
Residence: Inglewood, California
Lost his wife Shanda B. Strode (48) 2/1/2005
Cause of Death: Pneumonia

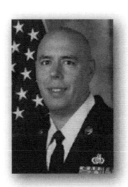

Contributing Widower: Master Sergeant Christopher Sweet
Career: U. S. Air Force
Resident: Navarre, Florida
Lost his wife, Technical Sergeant Jessica Sweet, (30) on 2/12/09
Cause of Death: Acute Myeloid Leukemia

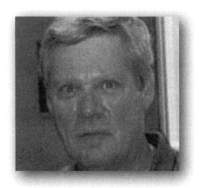

Contributing Widower: John Von Der Haar
Career: IBM/Siemens Administration Manager
Residence: Palm Coast, Florida
Lost his wife Mary (63) on 5/18/13
Cause of Death: Lung, liver and metastatic cancer

CHAPTER 7

Dating

The summer after Michelle died, I was still an emotional mess. I hadn't lived in San Antonio long, so my home phone rarely rang, and my doorbell never chimed. I was on anti-depressants for a month, and the doctor who prescribed them recommended that I see a psychologist, which I did in August.

At one point the psychologist asked, "What's keeping you from dating?"

For widowers, I've learned, that's a question with many answers. It's also a kind of litmus test, with the answers telling us many things about ourselves, including how we're recovering from the loss of our wives and how we feel about ourselves. In my case, when the psychologist asked that question, my first answer was, "That would be cheating, wouldn't it?" We discussed my feelings for a bit, and then she asked, "So what else is holding you back from meeting new women?" My second answer was as telling as my first: "If I don't get involved, I can't get hurt." So I was not only protecting my loyalty to Michelle, I was protecting myself.

And those were just my first two responses. I also wondered: Is it too soon? Where would I begin? Why would anyone be interested in me, a man married twice, one marriage ending in divorce, and the second in becoming a widower. Talk about baggage. And I thought my best years were behind me. I wasn't in the physical shape I was once in. No one widower is a poster child for dating angst, but I bet I came close.

And in my interviews with fellow widowers, all these issues were echoed. So in this chapter, we'll look at dating and developing new relationships, and we'll address those issues. We'll also examine a larger question: Is a new relationship something you need or want?

Of course, I did start dating. I'll get to how I arrived at that point in a bit. But first, let's look at other widower's experiences and sort through some important issues that can hold a widower back from a new, meaningful relationship.

Barriers

Many men doubt that they have the capacity to love again or that their hearts have room for both the loving memories of their late wife and love for a new woman. Widower Harold Moran hit the nail on the head for me when he said, "Having a love so strong and pure and then losing it left me wondering if it was possible ever again to have what was lost."

Plus, the memory of being a caregiver is a traumatic one, and the thought of being a caregiver again makes us hesitant. Following his experience as a caregiver, Eric Brown viewed a new relationship as a possibility of having to care for someone again until she dies. "That's a big issue for me," he admitted. "I would love again. I just don't know that I'm ready to take on the responsibility of helping someone else in the process of dying." Such thinking is on the minds of many. Being a caregiver once is hard enough.

And there is guilt. "I didn't date anyone for months after my wife passed away," said widower Steve Marquardt. "And when I finally did, I felt like I was cheating." Some men receive a kind of permission, which can be a blessing. Said widower John Heffernan: "Mary told me it was okay to be happy with someone else. And that such a day will come."

As I said, one of my major reservations was guilt over seeing another woman after my years with Michelle. But the psychologist I saw reminded me how I was married before I married Michelle. Even though my first marriage ended in divorce after twelve years, I must have loved my first wife at some point. The human heart is capable of loving more than one person, and to love again doesn't diminish or betray the love you once had. Also, my brother Dave asked me an important question: "If you knew Michelle would die after 16 years, would you still have married her?" Of course, I said yes. David's question taught me to draw circles around periods of my life. Having done so, I know I felt free to move on to the next.

Now we come to a delicate subject: What place should your late wife have in your life as you enter into a new relationship? A woman I know sought my advice when she discovered that her fiancé continued to write messages to his late wife on the Legacy.com website. It had been nearly ten years since his wife had died. One of the notes he posted said, "I still miss you dearly."

Professor Carr says that "Just because a man is reminiscing about his former life doesn't mean he loves his new girlfriend or spouse any less. But he needs to be able to integrate those two parts of his life. Most experts agree that holding on to memories of the deceased loved one is healthy. Looking at photos and even having imaginary conversations ('What would my late wife say about this?') can be a source of support and solace. Memories of a late wife should enhance rather than impede a widower's life."

However, she cautions that if these memories prevent a widower from fully engaging in his everyday life—things like dating, going to work, visiting with friends, and developing plans for the future—then such continuing bonds are a problem.

A new partner needs to understand that a previous relationship is part of the fabric of someone's life, Dr. Carr says. "Even if a widower or widow doesn't discuss their deceased spouse with their new partner, they still may wish to re-tell a story about how they had a difficult healthcare decision to make, a problem with a doctor, or a bad experience when traveling to the hospital. A new partner should be a friend as well as a love interest, and friends should be able to talk honestly and openly about almost anything, without fear of judgment or the withholding of affection."

Clinical psychologist Edward Zimmer explains that a type of emotional integration is essential for the widower to be able to love again. The widower needs to combine his memories, feelings and continuing connection to the deceased with his emotional experiences in his new relationship, and to see his loss as a part of his whole, new life. "He is a widower, but he could now be a second husband or stepfather. His loss is a part of who he is, and that loss should not be denied or otherwise split off from him." Zimmer says a widower's life with his previous partner should be recognized and accepted by his new partner, even if he chooses not to discuss it with her.

And once again we need to circle back to the importance of fully grieving. "A widower accomplishes this by allowing himself to grieve completely so it is psychologically unnecessary to split off or deny the emotional memories of his loss from his new emotional investment," Zimmer says. "If this grief process is stymied and the new partner is seen as a replacement for the deceased, as opposed to a unique person in her own right, the new relationship will be compromised by the unprocessed feelings of grief."

I believe you can not only love again but also do so differently. To address that belief, I co-wrote the lyrics to a song titled *Love You Different* with Rob Harris, Marcia Ramirez, and Kim Parent.

Love You Different

I have come to know
The heart can love again
Even after true love has passed into the wind
There's no need to explain
What you're going through
'Cause not long ago I lost an angel, too
I know you miss him
But I'll love you different
I won't replace him or want you to forget
You'll never love the same
That's not for me to change
I know you miss him
But I'll love you different

Even as we let them go
Part of them will stay
Woven deep into our lives and who we are today
That's something we can celebrate

BRIDGE:
So let me wipe your tears away, my beautiful friend
I believe they'd tell us it's okay to love again

Copies of *Love You Different* are available on iTunes. To inquire about availability, write herb@WidowersSupportNetwork.com

---

And as long as we're on the topic of music, a dear friend of mine, Nashville singer-songwriter Ken Harrell, wrote and recorded a beautiful song titled *Someone I Can't Live Without.* Among the song's lyrics: "I don't want someone I can live with. I want someone I can't live without." Ken's music helped me crystalize my reasoning for dating. I didn't want to be with someone because I *could*. For me, doing so would cheapen any hopes I had for a lasting relationship. Don't settle. Don't confuse a crush with true love. (You will find Ken's CD *We're All the Same* and his CD *Hope* on iTunes. I highly recommend both.)

During my research, I discovered that some of the women who entered into the life of a widower didn't want to hear stories about the deceased wife. They didn't want to see her picture (especially in the bedroom) or be expected to listen to stories about her. Rather, they often wanted to have a life with the widower absent anything that reminded him of his previous love. Likewise, some widowers become dismissive or even insulted if their new partners talk at length about their late husbands.

In my view, it is unfair for new romantic interests to expect surviving spouses to refrain from talking about their late partners. History can't be erased. Sure, you should not overdo it, and you need to be sympathetic to your new partner's feelings. But you shouldn't be expected to ignore, conceal, or gloss over what was likely to have been a significant portion of your life. We're talking about both parties being reasonable.

Professional life coach Patricia Fripp says that a new partner should recognize that "We are the sum of our parts." And because that's true, all that a widower experienced before meeting the new partner contributes to who he is and why his new partner is attracted to him. Included in those experiences is a measure of integrity: The widower didn't run away from an ailing wife but chose to serve as her caregiver.

Let's be sure not to candy coat this. If remembering a past spouse is a persistent problem, a couple should seek counseling or part ways.

A Sweet Story

I'd like to pause here and tell the story of widower Chris Sweet, a Master Sergeant in the U.S. Air Force, whom I have quoted before. Chris lost his wife, Jessica, who was also in the U.S. Air Force when she was diagnosed with leukemia after being deployed to Afghanistan. When she died, she and Chris had three children, ages 7, 5 and 2. Chris said he never thought he would get married again but that he missed having somebody there to take care of—and who would take care of him. "I was all set to be miserable for the rest of my life."

"I also thought somebody entering my life would force both my children and me to push any memories of Jessica out of our lives. It was important to me that my kids grew up hearing all the stories about their mother, what kind of woman she was, and also for Jessica's family to remain a close part of our family."

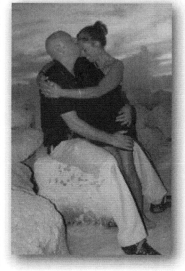

Chris wasn't looking for a relationship, but sometimes love just happens. Chris met Danielle Balmer (pictured here) at the Snowball Express, an event staged for children of fallen military personnel around Christmastime in Dallas. Danielle, a mother of two, had lost her husband, Ryan Balmer, a Special Agent for the U.S. Air Force when he was killed while serving in Iraq. Both Chris and Danielle openly honor each other's late spouses. At the time I interviewed Chris, both he and Danielle were wrapping up a T-shirt drive that honored Ryan and raised money for cancer research.

"I know how much Danielle grieves the loss of Ryan, and I know how much she loved him," says Chris. "I feel how bittersweet it is to watch as her children celebrate Ryan's birthday. I don't ever want to do anything to stifle their relationship with their father, and Danielle provides my children with the same support."

Chris and Danielle married on the Fourth of July, 2011. I haven't found a healthier example of how a widower and a widow manage their new unions.

Commenting on how both she and Chris are handling their relationship, Danielle said: "I think it's about love and respect. It's about the love that I have for Chris, and the love that he has for Jessica and their children. It's about the love and respect Chris has for me, and my love for Ryan, and for our kids. Just because our spouses are no longer here doesn't mean that they're no longer a part of our family or a part of who we are. Our grandchildren are going to know about Ryan and Jessica—about their grandma and grandpa that are not here. It's a matter of love and respect for everyone involved."

<hr />

We Have a Lot to Offer

When we finally decide we're ready to date, many of us look in the mirror and panic. We're older, rounder, and grayer—and sometimes crankier. We have obligations, baggage, and perhaps a bad habit or two. What woman in her right mind would want to deal with all of that, let alone snuggle up to it daily? Thankfully, the answer is many women would. And the odds are in our favor. Experts estimate that among people ages 50 and older, there are as many as three eligible widows for every widower. So there is no reason why a man needs to be alone. And this doesn't even take into account the number of divorced and never-married women who would be interested in dating a widower.

So what makes widowers attractive? Actually, many things make us uniquely attractive when compared to other men, and I've heard many stories of women who seek to date widowers. We have a history of staying in a marriage, even when times become tough. Unlike a divorced man who may feel resentful about his former wife, we may have loved our wife until the end. Many of us learned to be a caregiver, a skill that may come in handy later in life should a new wife take ill. And the experience of caregiving teaches us to be more giving and selfless—traits that many women welcome.

If you're anything like me, you'll become protective of the new woman in your life because you know tomorrow is not guaranteed. As a result, we may dote over a woman, and find ways to please her, even at a frequency greater than what we did with our deceased wife. However, we need to recognize that some women may feel suffocated by this devotion, especially if it's motivated by fear and anxiety. It's important to respect a new partner's boundaries and her preferences for how the new relationship unfolds.

Widower Otto Souder remarks how the widowed women he dated use to describe their deceased husbands as being a prince. "Well, I'm not," said Otto. And he's not alone, as not many of us could be described as being a Prince Charming. Some of us may have had difficulty during our grieving, and we still may be dealing with some lingering problems. And some of us may not have been particularly good husbands or caregivers for our late wives. Some might have been unfaithful. The pain of having lost one's wife does not transform a widower into a saint. But many of us have much to offer a partner. Take a look around. There aren't that many of us who stay single, especially if we're committed to finding a new partner.

How I Moved On

As I said earlier in this chapter, I had all kinds of issues that were preventing me from dating. Half a year after Michelle died, my grief had lessened from the pain I'd felt for months. I worked on building a social network, and I had a cadre of close friends. But loneliness for a romantic partner started to grow.

I decided to try dating. Some people might think that's too soon, but Dr. Carr points out: "Men who spent long time periods as a caregiver, especially to a wife suffering from terminal illness, may be ready to date much sooner. For these men, the loss of the woman they knew and loved might have come months before the actual death, as they watched their wives' personality, spirit, and even mental acuity slip away during her final days."

When I told my friend, Joe Dion, of my intentions, his response was, "I hope you're not looking for approval from anyone." I wasn't seeking approval, exactly. But there was someone I wanted to tell I was ready to date. That was my 23-year-old stepson, Jacques. I asked him if he believed I loved his mother. He said yes. Then I told him how I decided to build a new life for myself, a life that would include dating. He said, "It's about time." Those three words freed me from whatever guilt I still felt.

Of course, there are many ways to meet someone new: through friends, through church, through work, etc. I'd met Michelle through a blind date set up by my sister Patty. But, because I didn't have deep roots in San Antonio, I chose an Internet dating service. Guys, try it—especially if you're having trouble getting off the dime. Using a little bit of science to find compatible prospects doesn't take any of the romance away, and at least you'll be guaranteed to meet someone who is looking for someone.

After enrolling in eHarmony's program, I dated several women, a few of whom I found interesting and possessing relationship potential. Of course, eHarmony is just one of dozens of dating websites, many of which focus on particular communities. There is a dating website for just about every religion, age, and special interest.

As you might imagine, not all dating websites are created equal. Some are better than others. Such is the case with eHarmony.com.

How do I know this? My new wife, Maria, is a Ph.D. industrial engineer with a specialty in computer simulation. During her career, she came to know Dr. Thomas Parsons, a psychology professor that holds the patent for the eHarmony matching system. Dr. Parsons informed Maria that, according to a study, couples who get married after meeting on eHarmony exhibited a higher degree of satisfaction than couples that met by other means. Hey, it worked for us, and we couldn't be happier.

Two tips on using these sites: Don't exaggerate your qualities, and answer questions honestly. For example, I said I would prefer someone who shares my faith, but it wasn't a prerequisite. On the other hand, I refused to date anyone who smoked, drank heavily, or wanted to have children. If you're honest, you may be pleasantly surprised with the results. Also, don't be excessively picky. Limiting a search to only "slender" women may mean you miss out on someone who isn't slender but who shares all your hopes, dreams and values. Many men feel like a kid in a candy store the first time they check out Match.com. But the list grows much shorter if you filter it by "who would I realistically click with" and "who would realistically click with me."

One woman eHarmony matched me with was less than honest. At the time, I was 60 years old, and I asked her, "Why would a 48-year-old woman be interested in seeing a 60-year-old man?" After a pause, the woman slowly responded, "Well … I'm not really 48." So much for starting a relationship based on honesty. I actually continued to speak with her, though, realizing that she may have been compensating for male biases that would immediately dismiss a woman over 50. But when she told me her father was in the mafia, I took a pass.

I would counsel you to have some patience with the women you may date. Thank goodness, my wife, Maria did. In July of 2010, at the age of 60, eHarmony matched the two of us. We had our first phone call on a Monday night, and after maybe ten minutes she said,

"Okay, goodbye," and hung up. I was stunned. I told friends how it had been many years since a woman dismissed me so abruptly. After a few days, Maria sent me an e-mail which read, simply, "Any more questions?" I responded, "Yeah, what the hell happened on Monday evening's call?" Maria said she didn't think our conversation was going anywhere, so she decided to end the conversation. Thank goodness she had second thoughts. I invited her to dinner.

Aside from an instant physical attraction, the more I learned about Maria, the more impressed I became. Maria fled Cuba with her then-husband, a former political prisoner, due to persecution by the Cuban communist government. Once in America, Maria earned her U.S. citizenship, as well as an engineering degree with honors from the University of Miami, and later her Masters and a Ph.D. from the University of Central Florida as an industrial engineer. Maria retired a few years ago from the U.S. Department of Defense where she worked for 23 years.

When meeting a woman online, widowers need to be mindful that she may be a bit nervous. Men need to assure them of their honorable intentions. For our first date, Maria and I decided to meet at a restaurant, thereby preventing me from knowing exactly where she lived. Maria also told her brother where she was going, who she was going to be with, and what time he could expect her to check in with him following the date's conclusion. She made all of these preparations to ensure she felt comfortable and safe. Those widowers looking to date may wish to suggest similar dating plans until such time your new lady friend recognizes your intentions are honorable.

Another suggestion: Don't be in a big hurry to go for that first kiss. Maria says I scored points because I didn't try to kiss her goodbye in the restaurant's parking lot. By the time we had our third date, I knew our budding relationship had serious potential, which was a far cry from thinking that I would likely never love again following Michelle's passing. Was I ever wrong about that—not to mention grateful.

Our romance grew rapidly, and in December of 2010, I asked Maria to marry me. Our wedding took place onboard the Ruby Princess, somewhere between Athens and Venice off the coast of Italy in August 2011. Because of our deep religious beliefs, we later decided to secure the blessing of our church by being married at Maria's home parish in the Catholic Church. Our children served as our witnesses.

Where to Look

I discussed online dating sites earlier, but I'd like to add the experiences of other widowers on good places to find good partners. Widower Steve Marquardt joined Parents without Partners, which is also where my brother Don met his wife, Kathy, and they have been married for 31 years. Widower Norris Jergenson says he met women by attending his church's "GriefShare" sessions, and he joined a singles club.

Some of us widowers, especially those living in retirement communities or large residential complexes, may think dating someone who lives in our building or on our campus is convenient. Widower Doug Covert is a bit more cautious, however. He tells us; "In a condo complex, there are many committees one can serve on which may lead to some attractive introductions. Tread lightly. If a relationship doesn't work, then you'll need to deal with uncomfortable moments of seeing each other in the elevator or at the club house.

Sometimes, relocating to the right environment opens the door to new relationships. For example, in 2010, I relocated from San Antonio, Texas, to The Villages, Florida. While I didn't consider the prospects of meeting single women as a reason for moving there, The Villages is fertile ground for singles. I've even heard that the ratio of single women to men is 8 to 1. The Villages is a fast-growing, self-contained community located between Orlando and Ocala along I-75 and the Florida Turnpike. With a population of more than 120,000 and growing, not to mention more than 70 golf courses, The Villages is home to people from across America.

The Villages has long been known as a place abundant with single women. In fact, it is rumored that there is a group known as the Casserole Ladies who deliver casseroles to single men as a means of introduction. It always troubled me that I never received a casserole. (I got over it. Besides, I was watching my carbs.)

The lesson I've learned from interviewing many widowers and speaking to experts: If you're looking and not finding anyone, shake things up. This may mean Internet dating, joining clubs, or even moving.

Men Give Men a Bad Name

One obstacle you may face when seeking a new love is the women who have been hurt by men who give men a bad name. Unfortunately, there are men who don't respect women, or who repulse women by being greedy, self-centered, and shallow. The list I've heard from widows goes on and on.

One day while I was doing work for the Michelle's Angels Foundation, I received a request to contact a woman who lived in New Jersey. I'll call her Rita. Rita had been fighting cancer and had already undergone a double mastectomy and a hysterectomy, and she had begun both radiation and chemo treatments. When I spoke with her, a business professional and the mother of one son, she described how she had to wear her chemo pump at work because she wasn't able to take time off to go for her chemo treatments. She had no other means of income, which she desperately needed to care for her son. I asked if she had a husband, to which she responded: "I used to have one of those. He didn't like the way I looked after my double mastectomy." Rita's husband had abandoned her at the most difficult time of her life. I can't fathom how a man—and I use the term *man* loosely here—could have such an absence of decency and character and even consider abandoning his wife.

Women are the greatest gift to men. And men such as Rita's ex-husband should have a warning label tattooed on their forehead: "Beware: no redeeming qualities." And perhaps a skull and cross-bones tattooed alongside it.

The good news is, while researching *The Widower's Journey*, I found most men to be caring and dedicated to the love and union they shared with their wives. And usually, their dedication to their union became stronger when facing adversity. Such was the case during Michelle's thirty-nine month battle with cancer. That time turned out to be the most loving and caring years of our marriage.

I mention all of this because when you're taking the long look in the mirror, you need to ask yourself, "Am I one of those men who give men a bad name?" If you think you are, you might want to skip back to Chapter 3 and re-read the part about finding a new purpose in life—one that leaves those bad behaviors behind. I've interviewed many widowers, and I know some have engineered profound changes in their lives, so don't give up hope.

Predator Women

While we're on the subject of bad behavior, widowers need to be aware of the threat posed by predator women. Predator women are rare, but they still may present a significant legal risk to widowers. They have one main goal, which is to gain access to the wealth of widowed men, this according to attorney Diedre Wachbrit-Braverman, who says she has come across more than a few such women in her practice. Widower Jeff Gower experienced the pain a predator can inflict when he married his second wife just sixteen months after his beloved Susan passed away. "My new wife was doing everything she could to wipe Susan out of my life," said Jeff. Jeff divorced his second wife, but not before his substantial wealth was depleted.

Unfortunately, not everyone a widower will meet will have the widower's best interests at heart. Widowers may be in a fragile emotional state, so they need to go slowly in all things that they do, including dating. And if you are as fortunate as I was to find love and are considering marriage, be sure you protect yourself from the well-hidden intentions of someone less honorable than you. Consult an attorney and explore the benefits of prenuptial - and postnuptial - agreements.

Let me end this chapter by saying that just because it's possible to love again, it doesn't mean you'll necessarily want to, now or ever. My father is a case in point. Following my mother's death, most of my ten siblings and I encouraged my father to seek companionship. On my 35th birthday in 1985, my father called to wish me a happy birthday, and while on the phone he asked, "When are you going to marry?" To which I responded: "Just as soon as I am ready. When are you?"

My father, with a chuckle, said, "I'd rather have a cheese sandwich." I laughed, of course, but I also knew that deep down my father wasn't ready to move on, though my mother had died four years earlier. My father understood how most men would be happier with a loving partner, which is why he asked me about getting married. He was 70 at the time—exactly twice my age—and he lived to 77 without ever seeking another love.

CHAPTER 8

What about Sex?

F ar be it from me to give fellow men advice about sex. But there are a few issues worth mentioning. I'll keep it brief; this is the book's shortest chapter. Most widowers hope to re-establish a sex life at some point, and sex as part of a new relationship can be an important step in a journey to recovery. But sex may come with strings attached. In this chapter, we will explore some of the issues related to a widower's sexuality, including guilt, hurdles, and risks.

Are You Ready?

For some widowers, the thought of beginning a sexual relationship quickly is extremely tempting. This may be even more the case for widowers who abstained from the pleasures and joy of lovemaking during the time their late wife endured a protracted illness. And asking a man if he's ready for sex may be like asking a bird if it's ready to fly. But in many ways, a widower is starting over emotionally, so he's like a hatchling leaving the nest for the first time.

Allow me to suggest that a widower who hasn't dealt with his grief sufficiently isn't going to gain much relief through sex. Sure, satisfying your sexual desires is fun, but doing so while you're still vulnerable tempts mistaking sex for love (more on this later). It can start you in a misguided relationship, and then there's the worst case scenario: More than one widower I have interviewed has proposed marriage in the heat of the moment, only to regret it later.

Clinical psychologist Edward Zimmer cautions that "widowers may be caught off-guard by unanticipated feelings of grief when they engage in sex the first time since their loss. Such feelings are perfectly normal." But I'd add that it doesn't mean they're ready for a relationship. Zimmer also suggests that how one feels with a new sexual partner (at least in the early stages of the relationship) may be intimately tied to one's sexual relationship with their late partner.

Also, would adding sex to a relationship before you're ready harm the potential for a loving and lasting relationship? As you and your romantic interest begin to discover a mutual desire in one another, and if sex becomes awkward or a barrier, it's a good idea to take a break and talk about your issues. Facing them head on will help cut those strings, and it shows respect.

Are You Up To It?

As we age, we face some health issues that may affect our sexual performance; conditions including heart disease, diabetes, depression, low testosterone, and prostate cancer can hurt our ability to perform sexually, as can feelings of guilt. For instance, one in seven of us will eventually be diagnosed with prostate cancer, affecting not only our health and longevity but also our sexual functioning. And antidepressants, which many of us take to help us deal with our grief, can also cause erectile dysfunction (ED).

Fortunately, there are several great drugs to treat ED. Don't be shy about asking your doctor for a prescription—about 40% of men in their forties suffer some form of ED, and that increases to 50% of men in their fifties, 60% of men in their sixties, etc. The drugs, such as Viagra and Cialis, can seem like a fountain of youth, but take it easy if it's been a while.

Such talk reminds me of something widower Douglas Covert, Ph.D., told me. Doug was at one point concerned about having developed prostate cancer. When this happened, he considered castration. Why? Well, according to Doug, "When you take sex out the picture, things become much less complicated." True! But I'm still not ready for such measures.

We have all heard stories about men who die having sex. I know most men scoff during the part of the ED commercial when it says, "Ask your doctor if you're healthy enough to have sex." And you may be thinking, "What a way to go!" But be smart about it. ED drugs have many side effects, especially for men who already have heart conditions. Although these topics may be embarrassing, it's essential to discuss them with both your doctor and your partner. A few moments of embarrassment are a small price to pay for your health.

And speaking of embarrassment, here's another important pill to swallow: Be sure to ask your doctor to test you for sexually transmitted diseases. Your new partner should do likewise. Don't snicker if you're older. The incidence of sexually transmitted diseases has risen in lockstep with the increasing use of ED drugs.

It's also important for widowers to recognize that physical limitations can be opportunities. For some older adults, "sex" as they used to perform it is out of the question. But many widowers and their partners discover that they can have sexual relationships even without having sex.

"Sex is important but over-emphasized. Just holding one another, petting, and touching can be satisfying," says widower Aaron Seiden. Professor Carr tells us the data backs that up. "For older couples, especially those with physical health conditions, cuddling, kissing, petting can provide just as much satisfaction as intercourse. Couples may even grow closer as they develop their own repertoire that is physically and emotionally rewarding, yet at the same time recognize the partners' aging bodies."

Sex Versus Love

In my view, making love is altogether different from having sex. Professor Carr tells us: "It's important to come up with your own definitions of 'love' and 'sex' before having a new sexual relationship, and making sure that you and your new romantic partner see eye to eye regarding your desire for real love versus simply making love. Love making requires an understanding between partners, and the sharing they will enjoy together."

It is easy to get love and sex confused, especially for those who have not had a romantic relationship in many years. In his book, *The 3 Elements of Making Real Love: Sex vs. Making Love—For All Couples,* Darryl Y. Barron writes, "Don't be confused in thinking that a good orgasm means you have just made good love. It simply means you just had good sex by means of being stimulated physically and emotionally enough for you to achieve an orgasm." Dr. Carr adds, "Studies show that close physical contact and sexual relationships release chemicals such as endorphins, which may temporarily trick the brain" and make someone feel as if he is in love. "It is unfair (and dishonest) for sexual partners to promise each other love when in reality they simply see one another as a fun—and perhaps temporary—diversion from their grief," she says.

Barron adds that making love without expecting anything in return makes it more meaningful, "which in turn adds to the longevity of your relationship because sex alone is not enough to sustain a good long-term relationship."

Beauty fades. With each passing year, hairlines recede, waistlines expand, and virility declines. As a result, you may question whether you are even attractive to a new sexual partner. The answer is yes. It just means finding the right partner.

CHAPTER 9

Marriage

Before she died, Carolyn Covert told her husband, Doug: "Your life shouldn't stop. If you married again, it would show how happy our marriage was—that you'd like to try it again." Carolyn's feelings mirror my own. In a sense, I celebrate Michelle's life by living mine. It shows that the success, joy, and love that Michelle gave me in our sixteen years together made me secure enough to seek happiness despite her loss.

Several of our contributing widowers said that their spouses told them something similar. Their wives hoped their husbands would find a new life for themselves, even if it included finding a new love.

The story that touched me the deepest came from Carl and Patricia Jahrstorfer, which I discussed in Chapter 3. What I didn't mention is that Pat had said to Carl before she died that he should marry a woman who was younger than him; a woman who could cook and had more energy than she did. And because Carl was the last in a long line of Jahrstorfers, Pat suggested that his new wife should already have a son that Carl could then adopt. That way, the Jahrstorfer name would live on following Carl's death.

Women are wise, and they often know us better than we know ourselves. But whether or not you received your late wife's blessing,

I (obviously) believe marrying again doesn't compromise her place in your life. Though remarrying may be an issue for some widowers, it is one I hope I can help dispel. Beyond that, widowers need to approach marriage with several things in mind, and I'll go over those in this chapter. I'll also discuss when marriage may not be right, talk about alternatives to marriage that widowers may consider, and briefly touch on some financial and legal issues.

But first, let's do a little review. As I wrote in Chapter 7 about dating, widowers have much to offer a woman, and so they have much to offer a new wife. Some widowers have provided for an ailing spouse—a trial that develops character—and those who had long marriages show they know how to serve as a life partner.

I believe that the experience of being a widower, though painful, changes most men for the better. Their character is tempered by their grief, and if they seek the support of others—as many do and all should—they also learn a great deal about compassion. When I interviewed widowers, and they shared their heartfelt feelings with me, I was touched by the loving nature and tenderness most of them expressed. So I can say without reservation that the vast majority of the men I have interviewed would make wonderful spouses. In fact, I was so impressed that I set up a few of them with women friends. (Nothing has gelled yet, but let's give it some time!)

But don't just take my word for this. You may recall the story of Danielle and Chris Sweet, who lost their military spouses, and married and merged their families. When I was speaking with Danielle, I mentioned how I thought that I might be a better husband this time around. Danielle immediately agreed. Danielle said that before she met Chris, she had been speaking with a friend whose husband had been killed a few months after Danielle's husband, Ryan, died in Afghanistan. "My friend had met a guy who she had started dating who happened to be a widower. She said I needed to find myself a widower because widowers know exactly what I [she] was going through." Danielle quoted her friend as saying: "I can talk about

Tom [her deceased husband], and he understands. He talks about his late wife, and I understand." Danielle said, "Together, they 'get it,' and there are no ill feelings or competition." Danielle said that though she wasn't seeking a widower when she met Chris, she found that all of those things were true.

And widowers may have other emotional advantages. Professor Carr points out that divorced men often have lingering financial and custody battles that cause them personal stress, and that stress can't help but seep into their new relationships. Although widowers may be grief-stricken, they have fewer persistent stressors and don't have to negotiate often tricky arrangements with a former spouse.

Are You Ready?

And as I've mentioned, men, more so than women, tend to seek a new spouse and do so more quickly. In a *New York Times* article (June 1, 2006) titled "Widowers Are Eager for Another Whirl," the writer quoted author and relationship expert Susan Shapiro Barash as saying, "For men whose marriage ends only because of death there is often a desire to repeat the happiness they knew." Barash, a teacher at Marymount Manhattan College, added: "These men love being married, and they are good husband material. As the adage goes, 'when there is a death in a marriage, women mourn, men replace.'"

But what causes many widowers to rush to the altar at the first sign of compatibility? Rabbi Alexis Pearce advises all widowers to be patient. "Let time pass, even if you find someone perfect. Be suspicious of any urgency you feel to get remarried quickly; it probably isn't love," she says. "No one wants to suffer, but too much fear of pain or loneliness can lead us to rush into new unions that will not meet our expectations."

Pearce continues: "Grief tears the heart open, and often that means that we are more open to bonding deeply. But grief also unbalances family relationships and disrupts our sense of meaning and identity. When all of this is fresh, our judgment isn't what it will be in six months or a year." Rabbi Pearce recommends that "you bond, find companionship, spend time with people, get to know them, but hold off on permanent decisions until you feel your life would be livable with or without a companion." Rabbi Pearce's advice is sage and dovetails with Chapter 3, where we discussed putting your life back together. Each widower who is thinking about marriage should pause and be careful of making any rushed decisions that may be tough to reverse.

And consider that time can radically change our perspective—usually for the better. When I interviewed Norris Jergenson in 2011, he said: "I doubt that I will ever marry again. I think of Darleen every day." Norris remarried in August 2014. Once again proving, one should *never* say *never*.

Many widowers I speak to do not want to remarry because they have had enough of caregiving, and they don't want to bury another beloved spouse. They enjoy companionship and romance, but they aren't interested in being a nurse and caregiver again. Among younger men, this may not be an issue. But for people over 60 or 70, "till death do us part" is not merely a remote possibility. There needs to be a plan for when one or the other becomes sick or disabled. Who will be responsible? If one has children and the other doesn't, are the children ready to assume care of the new stepparent? If you aren't ready or able to think about this calmly, you probably aren't ready to remarry just yet.

During a meeting of the Widowers Support Network held in The Villages, Florida, one of the widowers reminded us that "relationships need to have a purpose." As when we take on any new endeavor, we need to know where we are headed. What is the end game? Companions? Lovers? Spouses?

Admittedly, some women will not continue to date someone who has taken marriage off the table. For some women and men, marriage is the ultimate sign of love and commitment. You'll have to judge each situation on your own. My advice is not to allow yourself to get boxed into marriage for the wrong reasons.

Another consideration before marriage is your children. Rabbi Alexis Pearce tells us: "If there are adult children, they will also be grieving for their mother and will need to form new bonds with Dad. This is a delicate process. When Dad rushes into a new relationship, children may feel shut out. They may feel Dad is betraying Mom. They may not have come to terms with Dad's needs for love and companionship; they may not trust or like the newcomer. But given time, if the new person is the gem you think she is, the kids will come to accept her and even be glad Dad is not alone."

Pearce says that a bereft and lost widower "may not care what the children think," but she urges them to "be patient and give everybody time. Be discreet, be gentle, and change things gradually. Have heart-to-hearts with children. The marriage will do better with family support. There's no rush. Change is hard for everyone, so go easy."

And I would add that you must remember that the woman you wish to marry may also have children who need time to accept any change. "Her children may need time to get used to the idea, and to decide you belong in their family," says Pearce.

Of course, remarrying isn't necessary for many men. Marriage is an important relationship, but far from the only relationship. Robert Schlieper, a widower from Buffalo, New York, began dating two years after his wife, Marian, died in 2004. The woman's name was Rosemary, and she lived in Long Island, New York. They would visit with one another often. "I was in love with Rosemary, but I just didn't want to get married." Robert and Rosemary broke off their relationship in 2009. Today, Robert lives in The Villages, Florida, where he has been seeing a woman for more than five years—with no marriage plans in sight. "I like living alone," says Robert.

Robert is a perfect example of the "living apart together" relationship that has become increasingly popular among older adults.

The two partners enjoy each other, spend most of their time together, and effectively act like a married couple. But they maintain their own homes and bank accounts as a way to enjoy the dual benefits of affiliation and independence. When Robert recently spoke about his life as a bachelor, he pointed out how his lifestyle doesn't lend itself to marriage. I applaud Robert's ability to recognize what is in his best interest. Widowers need to understand that not everyone needs to be married to enjoy a full life.

Discovering Joy

Over the past nine years, while researching and then writing this book, I had the honor of meeting many wonderful and caring men who were widowed. In some cases, I also had the privilege of meeting or becoming acquainted with the new women who entered their lives, such as Chris Sweet's new wife Danielle and others. One such couple was Bruce (Bud) Savage and his new lady, Kitty Woytovich. Bud and Kitty have known each other since grade school in Old Town, Maine. They reunited while attending their 65th High School reunion, again demonstrating how widowers never know when or even how joy may re-enter their lives.

Following are Bud and Kitty pictured sitting beside one another in second grade; and a second picture of Bud and Kitty today. Kitty jokingly writes, "We never dated. He never asked." Kitty adds, "We are now living 'Happily ever after.' " Today, Bud and Kitty are together and reside in The Villages, Florida.

<hr />

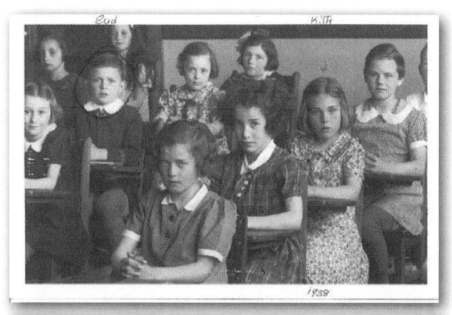

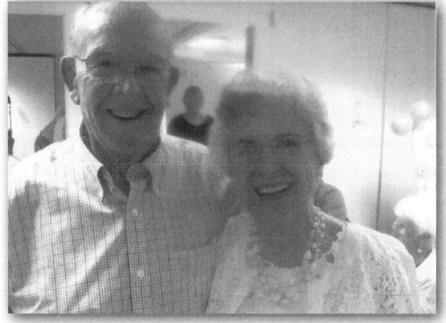

Finances

Part of putting your life back together before marrying again means having your finances in order. Finances are a touchy subject. Overall, people are more willing to talk about their sex lives than their finances. But being a widower has both positives and negatives regarding finances. I remember asking a woman who married a widower what she liked about dating and eventually marrying him instead of a man who had been divorced. I was taken back when she answered: "Widowers aren't sharing their paycheck or their pension with a former spouse." In a purely practical way, she makes an excellent point.

On the other hand, a widower may have a host of financial problems resulting from the death of his wife. He may have had his savings depleted by medical expenses; his credit rating may be a mess; he may have run up his credit cards, and he may have even declared bankruptcy. And the loss of a second income may mean he's having trouble paying a mortgage or making car payments. His job situation may be tenuous as a result of a long leave of absence.

Financial advisor Joseph Walsh, an expert at financial planning and strategies, says that a second marriage, especially later in life, can be much more complex than a first marriage. "Getting married when neither of the parties has assets, jobs, debts, or children is relatively simple. However, remarriage adds a new and often complicated, set of financial issues to consider. Children from a previous relationship, accumulated assets, accumulated debts, potential liabilities, and different styles of making financial decisions all influence how the money will be handled in the new relationship. Each partner may have very different views on how to handle money issues."

I think entering into a marriage with this kind of financial baggage can be a recipe for disaster. Surprise debts, especially, can cause a great deal of resentment. I talk about getting your financial house in order in Appendix I, and I recommend you take the steps outlined there before considering marriage. And in any case, before marriage, you and your partner should practice full financial disclosure.

Legal Considerations

Especially because a man may rush into a marriage after becoming a widower, it's important that he protect himself legally. As you can imagine, legal matters can be complex, and they vary from state to state. So I won't try to explain all the ins and outs (though more about legal considerations are in Appendix II). What I can tell you is that you need to see an attorney, and when you do, be sure to ask about prenuptial agreements, postnuptial agreements, elective share, and a new will.

Prenuptial agreement. A prenuptial agreement is especially important because you are likely to have many more assets than when you began your previous marriage. And prenups cover much more than just the protection of assets, so you should get legal help in drafting one. A prenup can also get into spousal support in case of divorce; it can protect spouses from being responsible for each other's debts; and it can make sure your kids from a previous marriage are provided for, among other things.

A prenuptial agreement can also protect you from disaster: the predator spouse eager to get her hands on your assets. This is the top legal problem facing widowers, according to attorney Diedre Wachbrit-Braverman, an expert on the subject.

Postnuptial agreement. According to MaritalMediation.com, "Postnuptial agreements are written agreements signed by spouses after their marriage to one another. So they are like prenuptial agreements, but they are entered into after the marriage takes place."

But why would a postnup be needed if you have already signed a prenup? There are various reasons to do so. For example, a postnuptial agreement can be of particular importance if the widower has substantial retirement or 401(k) accounts because federal rules dictate that the surviving spouse is the beneficiary of the retirement and 401(k) accounts unless that spouse specifically waives these benefits, according to financial advisor Joseph Walsh. A prenuptial agreement, if executed, fails to protect the widower because at the time a prenuptial agreement was signed, the spouse was not yet a "spouse." Should a widower who has remarried pass before his second (or third) wife does, she would be entitled as the beneficiary to the deceased widower's retirement and 401(k) accounts, regardless of who the deceased widower named as the beneficiary, including any surviving children from his first marriage.

Elective share. Nolo's Plain-English Law Dictionary defines *elective share* as "the portion of a deceased person's estate that the surviving spouse is entitled to claim under state law. In many states, the elective share (also called the statutory share) is about one-third of the deceased spouse's property. In some states, however, the amount the surviving spouse can claim depends on whether or not the couple has young children and, in a few states, on how long the couple was married. In most states, if the deceased spouse left a will, the surviving spouse must choose either what the will provides or the elective share."

Will. According to Marriage Missions International, "new wills are an absolute must so that each of you will know which possessions will be yours upon the death of the other and to formalize your wishes regarding any other separate or joint heirs. Be sure that your will mentions that a prenuptial agreement has been made."

Regardless of your situation, the laws that apply to your situation (federal and state) can be your friend or your enemy. If you have assets to protect, be certain to seek the services of a competent attorney who has experience in this type of law. Don't ignore it, naively thinking that nothing bad can happen in the future. Play it safe. You'll be glad you did.

CHAPTER 10
Helping Your Children

A s a widower, you know that you are not the only one grieving. Following the loss of your wife, pain is felt by many others, such as a mother, sister, neighbor, or friend. It can be just as intense as what you experience, and this is especially likely for children. Being the surviving parent of grieving children is another challenge, and sometimes it is the most difficult role a widower faces. You need to understand that role and help tend to your children's grief while you tend to your own. It may be especially critical for men who are fathers to young children.

In this chapter, we'll discuss how best to help your children. We'll cover communication, obstacles you may face, and how to handle questions or issues your children may have if you start dating.

Just as there is no single way to grieve, there is no single way to become a single, supportive parent. But I will propose one hard-and-fast rule: Be open. As we've discussed already, men who suppress their emotions hurt or permanently stunt their recovery. And experts tell us that as you deal with grief yourself, openly and honestly, you are also helping your children. So nothing is gained by suppressing or hiding your own recovery—in fact, that can be detrimental. Says clinical psychologist Edward Zimmer: "If the widower cannot allow for expressing and processing his own grief, then he will inhibit that process for his children. This unresolved grief will have emotional consequences for both of them later in life."

And if that isn't motivation enough, there is a silver lining to sharing. Professor Carr says the death of a mother can bring fathers closer to their children. "Women are usually the ones who make the phone calls and that the kids lay their hearts out to. Often a husband will just say, 'Talk to your mother.' But when the mother is gone, they may see a real increase in the level of closeness with their kids." That was the experience of widower Chris Sweet, who said playing dual parent roles was difficult, but it brought him and his three children closer. "I was close with my kids before, but we bonded further. It was a tough time for us, but I always made sure that we enjoyed our time together. We were able to laugh, and we had as much fun as we could have."

Communication

Few things in the human experience are as nuanced as communication. And generally speaking, we men not only don't communicate as often as we should, but we also miss the nuances. Widower Phil Carbone spoke for many of the widowers I interviewed when he told me he worried not only about the right way to speak about their mother's death with his children, a 25-year-old son, and a 23-year-old daughter, but he also worried about the timing and how much to talk about it. "I did my best at the time, but you never know the right way." But Carbone also knows the key to communication, which is simply keeping the lines open. "Sometimes you don't have to talk about it, but just doing things together will make a major difference." So just by being present, conversations about their mother often will open naturally.

Being present is particularly important for younger children. Dr. Carr says a widower "needs to reassure the young children that he is there for them, that he loves them and supports them, and that their new, smaller family is a united team. Young children need to be reassured that they are in no way responsible for the death. Some young children believe if they behave badly or act out, that it will make Mom or Dad 'go away'—whether through death or divorce. The most important thing the widower can do is provide a sense of safety, security, trust, and love."

That doesn't mean you shouldn't also start conversations, because sometimes kids need permission to open up. Dr. Carr says that some children may be afraid to open up because they don't want to upset their father. "It's not that they're trying to forget their mother; they simply don't know how to deal with the elephant in the room. Discussing death is difficult and painful, no matter how old someone is." She says some bereaved children hesitate to share their feelings of sadness and loss with their father, instead of feeling that they should be a source of support and strength. "It is important for widowers and bereaved children to recognize that both will need support. There will be good days and bad days for both, and family members should recognize that they could be a source of support to loved ones on their good days and can reach out to them on their bad ones."

Of course, how you support your children (or how children support you) varies based on the child's age. While adult children are often a source of support for older widowers, young children are often confused, traumatized, or scared by a mother's death.

Dr. Bruce Perry, M.D., Ph.D., of the Child Trauma Center in Houston, Texas, and an authority on brain development, writes, "Most children do not know what to expect following the loss of a family member or friend," and he encourages people not to be afraid to speak with the children. "When discussing this issue with children, be sure to use age-appropriate language and explanations. As the child gets further away from the event, he or she will be able to focus longer, digest more, and make more sense of what has happened. Don't be surprised if the child even acts as if the loved one is not dead or that Mommy will be coming back. It may take many moments of sadness for the reality of the loss actually to sink in for young children."

Widower Rutilo Flores was concerned about how his children were going to cope after losing their mom. "I wanted to be there for them. I told them, 'I won't try to become your mother. But I am here for you and you for me.' As it turns out, they both did great."

Dr. Carr cautions that "widowhood often does not change relationships. Some fathers were distant or remote when their wives were alive, leaving all emotional conversations and daily chit-chat to their wives. It's no wonder, then, that children may not feel comfortable reaching out to a father who was not engaged with them in earlier years, or who simply passed the buck to his wife when it came to family time." She notes that women are the ones children generally call for advice and who kids lay their heart out to.

That's all the more reason to give those quiet permissions to open up those conversations. It might be recalling a favorite expression the mother used to say or remembering a great family time you all had together. You can set the tone for communication.

Earnest Moran regrets that his children didn't talk about their mother more. "They didn't say very much to me. I don't know if they did with others. As it was, I felt very alone with my grief." Widower Rutilo Flores's two sons, ages 22 and 20, were eager to speak about their mother with him. Norris Jergenson tells us how his children don't bring up their mother's name often. They didn't display a need to speak of or about their mother. "I would love to have talked about her and wish they would have been willing to do so more often."

Not all communication is positive. Clinical psychologist Edward Zimmer says: "Some children who grieve express anger. Surviving children may have had a strained relationship with their mother and harbor anger that they will never be provided an opportunity to settle, now that she has passed away. At times, this is difficult. In the case of younger children, they don't possess the vocabulary or sophistication to put their anger into words, so they act out as a means of expressing their frustrations." Be sure to open up communication with your children's teachers and counselors, and let them know you want to hear about anything of concern.

Zimmer says: "In some households, the mother is the one who ensures the children stay in line, leaving the husband to be the good cop. With the mother's passing, suddenly, the good cop needs to be able to merge his deceased wife's role with his own. Children need structure, a set of double lines in the middle of the road to stay to the right of."

Dr. Carr says: "Parents of adult children often find that with the passage of time they realize that they genuinely like their children as friends and confidantes (although they, of course, have always loved their children). As children mature and establish their own lives, they may become their parent's peer, friend, and liaison" to a social or activity group.

Finally, if communication breaks down, you may need some professional help. "Some families may benefit from family therapy," says Dr. Carr, "as it gives them a safe space to have a conversation led and moderated by an expert. The therapist also may observe potentially harmful behavioral or communication patterns that the dad was unaware of."

The Importance of Friends

As a new, single parent with young children, you may need help taking care of your kids. And you may not have a family to rely on, so you may need to rely on family friends for support. It may be for simple things, such as providing rides for your children to school. Or it may be for bigger commitments, such as being with your kids when they get home from school until you get home from work.

Your first reaction, when such help is offered, might be to refuse it—certainly I've heard that from many widowers. As the reality of your new situation sinks in over the days and weeks that follow your wife's death, you may regret that decision. And while you may be able to get by, accepting help could make your grieving child's life easier. If there are people who have offered to be supportive that you have turned down, they may not ask a second time, and you'll have to reach out to them. Dr. Carr says that some widowers are so wrapped up in their own grief that they act in counterproductive ways, such as snapping at a well-intended friend or relatives. Dr. Carr notes that anger is one of the most typical reactions to loss, but it scares away the very people who could be the greatest sense of support to the widower. And don't forget, by accepting the help, you may be giving your friends a sense of purpose as they also grieve.

You may be lucky enough to have a bounty of offers from those who have offered to be there for you and your children. If so, here's a suggestion: Make a note of what their offers entail and then, when the time is right, share the list with your children and ask them if they would like to accept one or more of the offers. This process allows them to participate in their own healing. And Dr. Carr points out that it also teaches children (and their father) the importance of reciprocity. "No man is an island, and no one can survive on their own. By accepting support from a friend today, you may be called to provide help to that friend when he is someday in need. That's what relationships are about—give and take."

Traditions, New and Old

You might think that hobbies and activities aren't that important for family recovery, but they're part of maintaining and creating routines and carrying on traditions with your kids that help a great deal. They not only bring families together and provide much-needed normalcy in anxious times, they also can be a good way to remember your late wife.

My most stunning example of carrying on traditions comes from Steve Marquardt. He recalls how his wife, Merethe, died at home on Thanksgiving Eve. The next day, with help from her parents and his sister, Steve prepared a Thanksgiving dinner because he wanted the kids to have the normal routine. "I knew Merethe would have wanted that," he says. The next month Steve and his kids decorated a Christmas tree.

Dr. Carr says that some widowers purposely choose to have their kids participate in activities that their wife would have enjoyed, or to support her causes. "If a wife died of cancer, a widower and his children might start participating in charity walks or 5K runs to fight cancer. If she was a national parks advocate, they could contribute money or take over her volunteer work for her favorite park."

In my case, I wanted to find a way to stay close with my stepson, Jacques. When I founded the Michelle's Angels Foundation, I had to create a board of directors, and I asked Jacques to serve as a board member, which he continues to do to this day. I think it helped him deal with his grief, and it was therapeutic for both of us. I'm not advocating that every widower starts a not-for-profit and involve their children, but there are many ways a child could be involved with you in helping to remember.

Of course, you don't have to do something with your children that is directly linked to your late wife. Try coaching your kids' Little League baseball team or soccer team, or maybe serving as a Boy Scout leader. You'll be spending more time with your kids, and serving others is a great life lesson for any child to learn from their parent.

For those widowers who are still reluctant or not ready to volunteer, at least consider joining an organization that will provide opportunities for you and your children to do things together, such as Rotary Club or Kiwanis. They have programs in which children can participate. You can also find opportunities to deepen your relationship with your children by participating in church activities.

And, of course, children who mourn the loss of their mother can find strength from the teachings of your faith. If your children have not been introduced to a house of worship, after their mother's death could be an ideal time.

Dating: The Unique Challenges of Parents

Especially if your children are young, a new relationship after your wife has died can come with complications, not the least of which is your hesitancy to date because of your kids. In fact, I've found that one of the big reasons widowers fail to start dating is they think it will harm their children. Widowers worry their kids will have feelings of abandonment, or it may look as if a widower is not loyal to the memory of the children's mother.

Says Zimmer: "If a child or teen is acting out following the death of the mother or when the father begins to date or remarries, the behavior needs to be understood as a sign of emotional distress. Try to discover what your child is thinking. Bear in mind that a child may not know what is motivating the behavior, because we humans have thoughts and feelings we are not aware of." Disciplining the child in such a case would be a mistake, he says.

However, Dr. Carr says: "Widowers who have a good parent-child relationship are likely to have kids who are happier when they date, because they want their father to be happy. That's not to say they want him to be indiscreet or insensitive—dating before the funeral, for example. But after an appropriate period of time, most children embrace and even encourage their widowed parent's dating."

Dr. Carr says that some younger widowers may start to date or even remarry before they're ready because they are subconsciously searching for a helper and co-parent. "It's important to recognize, though, that all men are qualified to raise their own children," she says. "Just because they haven't been the primary parent doesn't mean they can't become one. Widowers may need to reach out for support, cut back on their work, or have a heart-to-heart with their children, acknowledging that he doesn't yet know everything that Mom knew. But loving fathers can get up to speed quickly with their parenting." They need to understand that so they avoid hasty or unwise romantic decisions.

Again, the answer is communication, and communication needs to start before dating begins. Tell your children how you're feeling, and remind them how you loved their mother and that dating in no way diminishes the love you had for her. You don't have to report to your children, but you need to respect their feelings by not being secretive. There is a good chance they will have questions about your new relationship, but are hesitant to ask, as they feel their questions may be intrusive. If you keep them in the loop, they'll feel freer to ask questions, and you can help head off any anxiety they may be feeling. For more information about how to communicate with children, visit The Fred Rogers Company website: www.fredrogers.org/professional/video/social-emotional/death.php

Dr. Carr has found in her research that older children could be helpful when their widowed parent wants to start dating again. "They often can help their dads and moms learn the 'rules' of contemporary dating and can be a source of advice and support, especially for those parents who are starting to date for the first time after a decades-long marriage."

CHAPTER 11

Keeping Her Memory Alive

W e widowers naturally seek a connection to our lost wives. It's healthy. In fact, psychologist Edward Zimmer says that connection not only helps us grieve, but it's also needed to help us form new relationships. So in this chapter, we'll talk about some of the many ways we remember our late wives, and we'll also talk about when memories can intrude on continuing our journeys to recovery.

Zimmer says that psychologists have surveyed groups of bereaved adults, asking the widowed about the ways in which they continued their connection to the deceased spouse. They found that a significant percentage of the widowed developed ways to keep their ties to their spouse, including through dreams and memories, by keeping some of their personal possessions, by taking on some of their behaviors and traits, or by visiting places that they had shared.

Matt Logelin did this in a big way. He wrote *Two Kisses for Maddy, A Memoir of Loss and Love*, a *New York Times* bestselling book (Grand Central Publishing, 2011). Matt lost his wife, Elizabeth, a day after she gave birth to their child, Madeline. *Two Kisses for Maddy* centers on Matt's marriage, the death of Elizabeth, and his experiences when raising his daughter. The book speaks to the two kisses Matt gave his daughter each evening—one from Liz and one from him. After Liz's death, Matt founded The Liz Logelin Foundation, which provides "support to grief-stricken young families in their time of deepest need." To learn more about the foundation, visit www.llf.org.

But back to the survey. Zimmer tells us how those interviewed reported: "The experience of continuing contact included sensing the presence of the deceased in some way. At times, the widowers would describe incidents in which they felt the deceased was trying to communicate something to them or in which they felt that the person had somehow intervened in their life in a positive and protective way. Others would simply describe an inner feeling of the person's presence.

"Sometimes there were inner dialogues that were reminiscent of conversations a widower had with the spouse. They might recount the day-to-day events of their lives, especially those events that the spouse would have been most interested in. Other dialogues were devoted to problem-solving; it seemed helpful for widowers to imagine what the spouse would have said in talking over a complicated situation. And sometimes they might communicate a need for help and protection, especially when they were facing situations such as illness or surgery."

Widower Phil Carbone chooses not to remember the day Lisa passed away. Instead, both he and his children have chosen to celebrate Lisa's life by remembering her birthday. "Even more importantly, Lisa wanted us to remember her in our minds and hearts."

One reason I established the Michelle's Angels Foundation was to continue Michelle's memory in my life. It was not only therapeutic for me to engage my energy and my business and marketing experience in this charity, it also led me to the establishment of a kind of ministry through which I can serve others.

Widower Harold Moran thought of a different way to remember his late wife, Connie. He says: "On our anniversary, Connie's family and I will get together to honor our marriage by baking Connie's favorite foods. It also provides a day of remembrance with our grandchildren. This year we will be using pumpkin grown in her garden." His youngest daughter, Heidi, even put together a cookbook of her mother's favorite recipes. What a great idea. Plus, Harold says: "On Connie's birthday, we all plant the same type of flower for her. Also, her organs were donated, so we've been to a memorial for her eyes and will attend another one for other organs."

Dr. Carr praised the rituals that Harold and his family celebrate. "After time has passed, and grief has faded, annual celebrations of our lost loved ones don't need to be somber," says Dr. Carr. "They can be ways to relive the humor, hobbies, and special traits of the lost loved one. Retelling funny stories and amusing memories is not sacrilegious—rather, it is an uplifting way to celebrate the life."

Widower John Heffernan buys an ad each year in the Boone High School Yearbook. His late wife, Mary, was a teacher in the school system, and he plans to continue buying ads until the 6th graders Mary taught graduate. John also takes out a tribute ad in Orlando's Conway Middle School, where Mary was a guest teacher, and has done so since Mary's death in 2013. To express his appreciation to those who cared for Mary, John arranges to have a pianist play in the main lobby of the University of Florida Health Cancer Center at Orlando.

Norris Jergenson remembers his wife, Darlene, each year by visiting the hospice located in The Villages, Florida, on the Fourth of July (the anniversary of Darlene's death). John also donates flowers to their church and spends the anniversary with his two children, sharing stories about life with Darlene.

Widower Rutilo Flores discovered a beautiful way to reconnect with his deceased wife, Raka. They married in Veracruz, Mexico, and Rutilo took their two sons, Ernesto and Ivan, to Veracruz so they could visit a park where Raka once enjoyed walking. After attending a church service nearby, Rutilo and his sons spread Raka's ashes in a park.

Walking in the footsteps of someone who has died can be truly therapeutic. My mother, Violet M. Knoll, died in 1981. Before she died, she attended the canonization of Saint John Neumann at the Vatican. As part of my wedding cruise with Maria, my new wife, in 2011, we stopped in Rome so I could walk in my mother's footsteps. It was a powerful moment for me, and I'm sure it was also powerful for Rutilo and his two sons to walk in Raka's footsteps.

"While visiting a gravesite is an important ritual for many, others may never set foot at the grave or cemetery," says Dr. Carr. "For some, the memories of their loved one are not linked to a piece of granite, but rather to a funny movie, song, or to a restaurant." She suggests that widowers celebrate the life of their late wife in the way that *she* would have wanted.

Other widowers will often continue to wear a piece of jewelry, such as a wedding ring, that makes them feel closer to their late wives. (Of course, that can become an issue when entering into a new relationship.) And some widowers have their wedding ring remade into a different piece of jewelry, another type of ring, or a pendant or pin. Of course, others pass the ring along to their children as an heirloom.

Here's an idea that may appeal to some: A company called LifeGem (www.lifegem.com) will take a bit of your loved one's ashes or a lock of hair, reduce it to carbon, and using heat and pressure turn that carbon into a diamond. And as the saying goes, diamonds are forever. The cost is about $3,500 for a quarter carat, and the diamonds can be made colorless, and in shades of blue, red, yellow, and green. Widower Jeff Gower had such a diamond placed in his Masonic ring. When people say, "What a beautiful diamond," Gower always says, "Perfect. It's man-made. Actually, Susan made it." Having Susan's remains compressed into a diamond was Susan's decision, he says.

Following the passing of his wife, Patricia, in 2012, widower Carl Jahrstorfer bought a unique ring from Expressions of Grief (www.expressionsofgrief.com). Carl's ring is stainless steel, with a black onyx outer ring. On the inside of the ring is inscribed the Serenity Prayer, which reads: "God grant me the serenity to accept the things I cannot change, the courage to change the things I can, and the wisdom to know the difference." The inscription also includes an image of a heart in two pieces. When others comment about the ring, Carl says, "It shows that while my heart has been split in two by the death of my beloved Pat, it is still open to receive and give love to someone else."

Widower Carl Jahrstorfer shared with me how he took his beloved wife Patricia's clothing to a seamstress and asked that it be turned into pillows. Carl refers to them as Love Pillows. What a clever idea. Each pillow was unique in its design, and the pillows were presented to friends and family members of Pat's, along with a personal message of remembrance about his beloved wife.

I was also touched and impressed by the story of Dean Troutman, who after the death of his wife, Dorothy "Peggy" Troutman, in 2010, vowed to build a park in her honor in Princeville, Illinois, where he and Peggy raised their four boys. The two had been married for 61 years. After spending about $300,000, he ran out of money. So to raise more money to finish the project he found sponsors and walked 700 miles one summer, at the age of 84. Today, the nearly six-acre park has a football field, a picnic pavilion, a baseball field, horseshoe pits, and a walking trail.

Social Media

For years, Americans relied on newspaper death notices to learn about someone's death. Now death notices are posted on the Internet, and the Internet provides some wonderful new ways to honor the deceased. Through memorial websites, we are now able not only to find the obituary of a friend or family member quickly, but also to see photos, read tributes, and even watch videos. Plus, we can communicate with survivors of the deceased by leaving a message online. In many cases, we are even able to participate in ongoing dialogues about the deceased and, in some ways, with the deceased. These sites include www.ForeverMissed.com and www.Legacy.com. With some of these, the service is free, or a basic page is free, with premium versions available that allow everything from private pages to background music (costs usually start around $50 a year).

Says Illene Cupit, a professor of human development at the University of Wisconsin, Green Bay: "When you go to a wake or sit shiva, if you're Jewish, you sit and talk about the person. You make sense out of what happened. And people are doing that now on social media." But what makes social media different, notes Dr. Carr, is that it may encompass a much wider net of friends and acquaintances than we might encounter at a funeral or eulogy. Bereaved family members may read about stories from their loved one's former colleagues or high school classmates—people we couldn't possibly know, in many cases. These new stories and perspectives provide entirely new glimpses into the person we thought we knew so well, and they can help us feel closer to our now deceased loved one.

Widowers Support Network (www.WidowersSupportNetwork.com), which I started, offers registered widowers the opportunity to honor their deceased wives by posting their picture along with a short story about the woman they loved. Registration is always free. We also post remembrances of the wives of this book's contributing widowers annually during the anniversary month of their passing. Social media and the Internet enable family and friends—including those who may reside at some great distance—an easy way to participate in the collective remembrance of a deceased family member, neighbor, colleague, or friend.

However, sometimes social media or the Internet can hinder a survivor's ability to move on. For example, you can set too many updates to remind you of special days in your relationship. The important thing about social media, says Dr. Carr, is to control it rather than let it control you. Dial back if it gets to be too much.

How Far Is Too Far?

Widowers need to be reasonable in maintaining their deceased wife's memory when they are in a new relationship or remarry. How do you gauge what is reasonable? A good way is to reverse roles and think what you would find awkward or intrusive if it were your partner remembering her late husband. Be careful of the time and place you mention your late wife. For example, if you take your new partner to a restaurant that happens to have been your deceased wife's favorite restaurant, there is no need to mention that over appetizers—or ever.

Never compare your deceased wife in any way to your new partner.

Then again, if referencing an event that took place during a former marriage, you should feel free to raise the name of your deceased wife without feeling like you have to tiptoe around it.

If the new person in your life is sensitive (not to mention mature), she will recognize the conflict you may be experiencing as you attempt to balance the memories of your deceased spouse with your feelings for your new love. She will embrace your history and allow some latitude as you juggle emotions. "And this understanding cuts both ways," says Dr. Carr. "Many widowers will be dating widows (or divorcees) who still have strong emotional ties to their late spouse. Sharing these memories together may actually strengthen, rather than threaten, your relationship."

CHAPTER 12

How Society Can Help Widowers

W e've now traveled together through a widower's journey. Hopefully, from my personal experiences and the advice from other widowers and our experts, you can find your way back to happiness with fewer false steps, and with optimism and confidence for your future.

As I've shown throughout this book, we widowers bear the loss of our spouses harder than do widows, both physically and psychologically, and in many ways, the deck is stacked against our recovery. This is because women tend to handle grief better than men. Of course, we're not asking for pity, but throughout the book, I've identified problems that should be addressed. So in this final chapter, I'd like to discuss how society can build a smoother, straighter road for widowers to travel on their way to recovery. If you've ever attended a marathon race, you know that not only are there crews of people along the long route handing out drinks and food, there are emergency medical technicians ready to help those who stumble, and the course is lined with fans yelling encouragement and support. Imagine how much easier our widower's journey would be if it changed from a lonely road to a marathoner's course.

As widowers, we can personally make this road easier for other men who have lost their wives, and we'll discuss how to do that. But we can also be advocates for societal change, which is one of my personal missions and one reason why I wrote this book. Society needs to understand better the emotional load widowers carry and be willing help them shoulder that load. That often means understanding the dead-end men are painted into emotionally, and being brave enough to help widowers—even when it's not obvious that we need support.

Every segment of society owns a piece of this pervasive, pernicious problem. That starts with our friends, our neighbors, and even our families. It continues to local mental health agencies, to employers, to houses of worship, and on up to federal agencies. No one gets a bye. My experiences and my research have shown that all of these parties have, to a degree, ignored the needs of widowers.

In my research, I have been heartened by what I see as a growing understanding of the plight of widowers in some quarters. But change is coming too slowly. Society needs to change. No longer should the 2,700,000 men who carry the label "widower" be left to largely heal themselves.

How We're Raised

I had never thought about the straightjacket that society laces men into until I encountered obstacles upon becoming a widower and interviewed so many other widowers who felt the same constraints. What has society created? We're in the 21st century, and yet our culture clings to this idea that men should always be tough, stoic, and able to recover from even the most painful of periods in their lives by simply sucking it up. And that they should feel ashamed for showing emotion or vulnerability, or for asking for help.

This starts in childhood, and as Aristotle said, "Give me a child until he is 7 and I will show you the man." The three most destructive words a boy hears are, "be a man," according to coach and former NFL player Joe Ehrmann, as quoted in the 2015 documentary *The Mask You Live In*. The film explores the root cause of a societal problem. It's an affecting piece of work, and describes itself as following "boys and young men as they struggle to stay true to themselves while negotiating America's narrow definition of masculinity." It starts with how many parents instill these standards of masculinity.

Professor Carr says that men, especially those born in the 1930s and 1940s, were raised to conform to what scholars call "hegemonic masculinity." This masculine "ideal" refers to the clusters of behaviors and feelings that men are expected to embrace or avoid. Some of the key elements are being strong, silent, unemotional, and dedicated to their careers (often at the expense of time with their families). Men learn things such as "boys don't cry" and are told to "man up" at the first sign of vulnerability or indecisiveness. Many also are raised to believe that "real men" are always interested in and ready for sex. Simply turn on the television or go to a Hollywood movie to see countless images upholding these expectations.

But few men actually conform to these expectations, and breaking from these expectations often comes at a cost. Boys and men may be ridiculed for showing signs of emotion or sensitivity. And at the same time, trying to conform to these unrealistic (and, frankly, ridiculous) expectations can cause men to feel anxious or trapped. And those feelings become even more overwhelming once a man is grappling with a new role as a widower.

And the media don't help things. From television shows to movies, the treatment of widowers rarely addresses widowers' issues in constructive ways, and often show that being a widower isn't such a bad deal. Take *The Courtship of Eddie's Father*, a sitcom from the 1960s. Eddie's father was a widower played by actor Bill Bixby, who was a little morose, true, but had his act together, plus a great housekeeper and an endless parade of attractive women to date. Fred MacMurray had the same situation in *My Three Sons*. And Mel Gibson practically built his action-hero career on exacting vengeance from being a widower—not exactly a healthy way to deal with loss. He did it in the Middle Ages in *Braveheart*, during the Revolutionary War in *The Patriot*, and as a cop in *Lethal Weapon*, 1 through 4. *Sleepless in Seattle*, though, did a nice job of showing widower Tom Hanks dealing with sadness and awkward dating situations. So maybe the tide is turning.

As we saw earlier in this book, widowed men often are expected to get back to work immediately and to put on their best game face at the office. I know that was my experience when I returned to work just ten days after Michelle's passing. And many of the widowers I interviewed had similar experiences. These expectations are all the more destructive to men who are fathers of dependent children; taking time out to mourn may mean the loss of wages to support their families. Other widowers are reluctant to reach out for help—whether they need a shoulder to cry on or help with preparing meals—because asking for help challenges the ideal of masculine independence. But as Dr. Carr explained earlier in the book, the most important thing in determining how well a widower adjusts to his new life is the amount of support he receives from others. No man is an island, nor should he be.

The challenges that widowers face when they dip their toe back into the dating game also can be intensified for men who can't free themselves of outdated notions such as men should always be interested in dating, that they should be the leader in the relationship, and that they should always be ready for sex. Widowers who are still grieving the loss of their beloved wives are simply not ready to start dating (never mind having sex)—even if well-intended friends keep telling them to get back in the game. Men who say that they're simply not interested in a romantic relationship yet may have their masculinity questioned.

What can we do—as individuals, parents, teachers, professionals, and even policy makers—as we work to build a society that supports widowers? First, at the individual level, we can be mindful of the stereotypes we hold and think about the harm in holding such beliefs. Have you ever said under your breath, "don't be such a sissy," or "gee, what a wimp" when a man showed grief or confusion? Have you ever thought that "the man should wear the pants in the family"? If so, then recognize the stereotypes you may be carrying around, and take conscious steps not to perpetuate them in daily life.

Second, if you are a parent or grandparent, think about the message you send your sons and daughters, children and grandchildren. Do you praise the boys for their strength and the girls for being pretty? If you need a cup of coffee, do you assume that your daughter rather than your son should fetch it for you? Sexist notions seep into our lives in subtle and pernicious ways. In reading this, did you first think, "raising the kids was my late wife's job"? If you answered yes to any of these questions, you are unwittingly contributing to a culture that silences and entraps both men and women in outdated and harmful gender roles. You can turn this around by teaching both boys and girls to hone their skills in cooking as well as money management, by encouraging both boys and girls to talk about their feelings when upset, and by letting them know that fear and sadness are emotions they need not be ashamed of.

Dr. Carr notes that human relationships are based on reciprocity—you help me, and I'll help you. You can show your kids by example that being the gracious and grateful recipient of someone's advice or support today means not only that you may pay back the favor tomorrow, but also that you will pay it back with interest. And you can show them that receiving help is not a sign of weakness; it's a sign that you are a human being who values others and will ultimately provide them support when needed.

Take That Step

The first overture to a widower can be the toughest. Dr. Carr recommends that well-wishers who don't know what to say to a widower simply ask the widower about the deceased, and let them share a memory. You know your wife has died, so it's no great surprise if someone raises the subject of her death with you. Let widowers talk, and don't let your fear of death get in the way of having a meaningful conversation." Dr. Carr went on to say: "Whenever people see or experience anything for the first time, they're not sure what to do. They don't have a roadmap. So the first time a young assistant sees his or her older boss cry, they simply may not know what to do. It's hard to get things right when we don't have experience in dealing with such matters. Nerves can get the better of us."

Dr. Justin Denney of Rice University believes people feel especially socially awkward when they see older male figures in positions of power and authority show vulnerability. And as I know from experience when I was virtually isolated in my grief at work after Michelle's death, acknowledging the vulnerability of a boss is something people are afraid to do. I recall late on my first morning back at work after Michelle's death, and while seated at my desk at the bank's headquarters in San Antonio, with my office door open, one of the bank's human resource officers entered my office. He appeared to be surprised to find me lost in thought with tears in my eyes. Not knowing what to say or do with a grown man crying, he immediately turned and exited my office, closing the door behind him. Perhaps if I was a widow instead of a widower, he might have taken a seat and offered a kind word.

Thank goodness my colleague Enrique Lerma summoned up the courage to drag me to dinner, as I related back in Chapter 6. I encourage you to take a leap of faith as Enrique did; matters of grief and recovery trump work and social hierarchies. Trust me on this.

Family, friends, neighbors, and colleagues need to be more diligent in their efforts to comfort and help widowers. I hope from reading this book you will have gained a greater understanding of what a widower goes through and that the knowledge will motivate you to be persistent.

Never leave a widower alone for too long. Call him regularly, even if it is just to say "I'm calling to take your pulse—you know, to be sure you are okay and to remind you that a lot of us care about you." Believe me; it means a lot to a widower. Even nine years later, I can tell you who checked on me and who didn't.

If a close friend loses his wife, be sure to continue to include him in all of the social gatherings he would have been invited to if his wife were still alive. Many men have told me how they had been excluded from social events following the passing of their wife.

Dr. Carr suggests that if you know an older widower, perhaps one who lives alone nearby, check on him both before and following a storm or heavy snowfall. Ask if he has enough medicine and food to get through the inclement weather. That simple expression of concern and recognition will go a long way toward building a bridge.

Man-to-Man Support

During the 2016 Republican presidential primaries, Ohio Governor and presidential candidate, John Kasich would routinely ask at campaign stops, "Anybody here lost a spouse?" According to an ABC News report, at a campaign stop at a VFW post in New Hampshire, a man spoke up amid the silence. He had been married 45 years before his wife passed away. Kasich then asked, "Anybody ever invite him to dinner? We gotta be a community. We gotta be neighbors. And I'm gonna try to get ya a dinner date."

I couldn't agree more, and to echo Kasich, we widowers need to be a community. I've spoken earlier about the importance of support groups and of contacting other widowers through various organizations. I'd like to take that a step further and suggest that even after you are through, or mostly through, your own widower's journey and may not need the aid of such groups, attend meetings anyway. Your own experiences will be even more valuable now that you've traveled your widower's journey ahead of other widowers in the group and can share with them your experiences, much as I've shared my own experiences in this book.

Now let me suggest a step beyond that: Form a widowers group yourself, perhaps through your church or a volunteer organization. In my experience, it just takes a group of men together and a couple to share their stories to get the ball rolling. And even if not in a group, reach out to a widower and take him out to dinner or a beer, even if you have to pry him from his shell.

How Society Needs to Change

A week after Michelle's death, I received a package from a leading life insurance company that included the proceeds from Michelle's life insurance policy. Additional materials were enclosed that were intended to encourage me to invest the proceeds in one of the company's annuities. But there was one major flaw in the materials: The insurance company's glossy promotional folder pictured a woman on the cover. The woman appeared lost and alone—a new widow. Because I had worked in senior marketing positions, I recognized how the insurance company's materials were designed to be received by a new widow, not a widower. While the information was useful, it was a reminder that society is geared to cope with the needs of widows.

I get it that such treatment is based on demographics. As Dr. Carr says, the insurance company's gaffe wasn't meant to hurt or dismiss widowers. If we look at the population of age 65+ people, there are three times more widows than widowers. But that doesn't justify the lack of understanding society affords widowers. The actions of the insurance company is just one more example of the void that exists. Dr. Carr says, "it carries two powerful and potentially harmful messages: Men aren't widowed, and if they are, they are strong enough to cope with it on their own. Both of those assumptions are clearly false."

Now just think of how that treatment of widowers is magnified throughout all levels and facets of society. As I've discovered from my own experience and from the experiences of the dozens of widowers I've interviewed, widowers feel ignored by the companies they work for to the churches they attend to the mental health and medical communities they visit. I'm going to lay the responsibility for problems that many widowers suffer at the feet of those institutions. Those problems include anger issues, loneliness, depression, alcoholism, drug abuse, and suicide. The problems include financial woes from losing a house to bankruptcy. And these problems don't stop with the widower but affect the widower's family as well.

Could the insurance company have designed its folder to include widowers, both in images and in the text? Certainly. And in retrospect, I should have dropped a note to their marketing department at the time. Since then, though, I have been nudging and cajoling and sometimes demanding that widowers be acknowledged by many institutions that ignore us.

Collectively, we widowers can help change how we're treated by institutions of all types. I believe if we raise our voices together we can change how society acknowledges and treats us. And, especially if you're in a position of influence, you can help steer policies. Certainly, there is no lack of widowers in such positions.

Consider businesses. We need local and federal policies and practices that help men and women juggle work and family when they're young, which will then prepare them to take on the tasks that may go undone when their spouse dies. Offering paid parental leave and family leave when one needs to care for an ailing parent sends a strong message from an employer (or the federal government) that one's capacity to work is based on one's family demands, just as one's capacity to support a family financially is intricately tied to the other demands one has. Workplace policy could also offer a generous bereavement leave, if needed, while employee assistance programs should provide grief counseling.

Good Economics

Just as it is in our nation's best interest to help the unfortunate and our wounded veterans, it is also in our nation's interest to assist widowers. The sheer number of baby boomers who will soon be widowed is sure to increase the burden on American taxpayers. Dr. Carr points out that our population is aging. By the year 2030, one in five people will be over the age of 55, and older people are more likely to be widowed. "The fact is, women are much more likely to be widowed than men. But in raw numbers, there are going to be many more widows and widowers who are going to need services."

The financial costs of grief and loss are difficult to quantify, although some organizations have attempted to do so. The Grief Recovery Institute Educational Foundation has placed a price tag of $75 billion on the annual cost of grief in the workplace. In a study, the Foundation predicted the cost of eight major grief incidents—from the death of a loved one ($37.5 billion) to divorce ($11.1 billion) to pet loss ($2.4 billion).

The challenges facing America's widowers represent a significant current and future financial cost to both taxpayers and industry. By addressing widowers' needs before they turn into physical or mental health issues or unnecessary lost time at work, we are not only sparing widowers from unnecessary suffering; we are also saving society money. So we desperately need a deeper understanding of widowers' situation and the need to shore up the availability of resources, programs, education, and active compassion for widowers.

There is progress on this front, make no mistake. I am particularly heartened by the growing men's studies field, often referred to as Men and Masculinity. This is an academic field of research that's been in existence only since the 1970s, and it examines men's traditional and changing roles in society. There is a Center for the Study of Men and Masculinities at Stony Brook University founded by Professor Michael Kimmel, who is a leader in the field and the founder and editor of the academic journal *Men and Masculinities.*

I spoke with Kimmel, and he says that when it comes to studying gender and aging, "90% of the material is about women. Men are almost completely invisible." He laments that while funding for women's issues has risen, funding for men's issues hasn't. And he says that when it comes to helping men, men are often their own worst enemies. "Men supporting other men, and men being emotionally caring for other men, is often seen as a sign of weakness," or it's seen as a sign of homosexuality. "Homophobia isn't just damaging to gay men; it's damaging to straight men as well," he says. That thought is echoed by Dr. Denney of Rice University. "By not supporting each other during trying times, by not allowing each other to grieve, men discriminate against each other."

So, as comic strip character Pogo once said, "We have met the enemy, and he is us."

But Denney sees a silver lining that comes from our society's focus on gender equality. "We tend to think about gender equality as how it will help women—for example, working for equality for women who make less money than men, even though they have the same job and the same background and experience. It strikes me that gender equality should help both men and women. If we can figure out how to say that women are just as intelligent as men and encourage more and more girls to pursue engineering and other sciences, then why can't we figure out how to say, 'Hey, men, like women, are emotional creatures and need help and support in trying times'? And that it doesn't make a man less of a person. I feel like the system is in place, but it's a matter of concentrating on how gender equality is good for everyone, men, and women."

If like me, you've finished your widower's journey and feel motivated to help widowers generally, I encourage you to become a crusader for widowers. I'm always trying to identify ways in which society fails widowers and seeking remedies for them, and I'm open to suggestions. But here are some things I've identified that are within our grasp and would go a long way toward helping the crusade.

Employers:

- Help members of your staff who are widowers or widows by offering free counseling and support. Companies with employee assistance programs should make sure the programs have channels for widowers and widows.
- Provide employees suffering from a family loss—be it the loss of a spouse, a child, or a close family member—more than the standard three to four days' bereavement leave or more flexible leave time.

Governments:

- Sponsor an event for National Widowers Day (get details at www.nationalwidowers.org), maybe by hosting a reception for widowers and widowers alike.
- Team up with local media to air public service announcements around major holidays encouraging the public to reach out to any widowers and widows who are celebrating the coming holiday alone.
- Designate an advocate to address the needs of the community's widows and widowers.

Houses of worship:

- Host grief counseling sessions and be proactive about inviting widowers.
- Host a monthly or quarterly religious service intended to recognize the widows and widowers in your congregation, and use the service to address their needs.
- Host a service to remember the spouses that have been lost, including a display of photographs of the deceased spouses.

Service providers:

- Retirement communities and senior housing complexes need to become aware of the unique challenges facing widowers and address them seriously with programs and services.
- Retailers and service providers need to ensure that their sales and marketing collateral materials are not biased towards widows or ignore widowers. Including both isn't a hard change to make.

This is my crusade, my ministry of sorts, and I'm always looking for recruits. If you're unsure how you can help, please feel free to contact me through my website. I consider all widowers my brothers, and our brotherhood can accomplish great things for our fellow men.

Epilogue

One can't help but be changed by a journey, and our widowers have some advice, with the benefit of hindsight from their journeys, that I thought was worth sharing. At the same time, in this epilogue I'd like to finish the stories of a few of our contributing widowers' journeys by giving an update on how they are doing.

The common theme of their advice is that losing their wives knocked their lives off the path they had envisioned for themselves and that ultimately finding a new path—often after some false starts—was something they didn't accomplish alone. They found their way with the help of many, including family, friends, neighbors, and counselors, and by attending meetings hosted by grief organizations. They realize that their late wives will forever be part of their lives and that keeping their wives in their memories is okay.

We learned from widowers like Quentin Strode (age 55) how most men are able to move on with their lives over time, including discovering love again. Quentin found love and married Sylvia Sanchez Strode in 2010. "I have moved forward, but the loss of my late wife, Shanda, still haunts me to a certain extent. And even though I married a wonderful woman, my late wife has a special place in my heart. I still think fondly of her daily."

Phil Carbone (62) showed us that recovering from the loss of his wife called for a lot of work. That being said, anything worth having is worth working hard for. "I have worked to save myself; to strengthen my relationship with my great children (and grand-children); to connect with my friends, old and new; and to build a life with my wonderful new wife, Marcia, and her children. I came close to giving up, but I am so glad that I didn't quit on myself or them." Phil and Marcia live outside of Buffalo, New York, and are building a retirement home in Florida. "I am not the same man," says Phil, "But I have *myself* back in a way that is meaningful and happy."

Several widowers said that in retrospect they were surprised how important attending grief groups was to their recovery. Norris Jergenson (75) attended GriefShare's series of meetings twice, while Bud Savage (86) was so impressed with GriefShare that he became one of its instructors. Paul Dispenza (60) attended GriefShare and later told us that he wishes he had done so immediately following the death of his wife, Melissa, instead of waiting two years. Today, all three men are doing well. Both Norris and Bud have found love again and live in The Villages, Florida. Paul is focusing on raising his two children, and he continues to work at a family restaurant in Amherst, New York, where he and Melissa first met.

John Von Der Haar (71) works part-time at a marina on Florida's Atlantic Coast, still dealing with his grief and the loss of his beloved Mary.

Eric Brown still lives in San Diego, where he serves as a financial advisor.

Otto Souder also rediscovered love and remains a resident of The Villages, Florida, where he is very active—which includes being found on a dance floor from time to time. Gary Secor (68) continues to serve as an independent representative for SalesForce.com and has started dating. Meanwhile, everyone's favorite postman, Aaron Seiden (91), and his wife are retired and spending their winters in Florida.

Colonel Brian Jakes (76) continues to serve as the CEO of a health education organization. He has remarried and resides in Mandeville, Louisiana.

Contributing widower Ralph MacNiven (69) and his new wife reside in the Naples, Florida area, where Ralph continues to operate an insurance agency. On the West Coast, Steve Marquardt (63) remains employed and is married to the founder of the Pancreatic Cancer Action Network (PANCAN), Pam Marquardt.

Rutilo Flores (60) continues to live in the Chicago area, where he has attempted to move on with his life. "I had no choice," he says. "While Raka was alive, she was my advisor, my best friend, my soul mate. I cannot hear her voice now, but when I am facing a situation, and I have to make a decision, I can sometimes feel her presence and take her advice in the way that she would have done would she have been physically present." Rutilo advises other widowers: "Close your eyes and put yourself in God's hands and let God guide you. For some reason that you would not understand, God put you through the loss of your wife, but He will help you to move forward. I believe that God has a plan for each of us. You have to carry on and make that plan come to life."

"I can't imagine how my life could be much more different now than it was before," says Rod Hagen (57) from Palm Springs, California. Rod lost his partner, Larry, after 34 years together. "I changed everything from my job to my house; I even changed my appearance, and it was all liberating." Rod adds: "Be kind to yourself. Be patient. Understand that an overwhelming feeling of grief may manifest at the most unexpected moments, especially in the first year. Allow yourself to feel that grief, even if it means crying in the frozen food section of the grocery store because some silly song started playing on the PA. Consider trying things you've never done before, even if you do them alone." Rod has discovered love and is in a new relationship.

Jeff Gower (59) advises all widowers: "Remember, we are not alone. Wherever we are in our life's journey, we arrived with the love, help, and support of many. And we should trust those friends with helping tend to our fragile selves, a bit like we trust a good doctor or counselor."

Earnest Moran (77) is doing well, has remarried, and is living in the Phoenix area. His semi-retired brother Harold Moran (66) continues to reside in Upstate New York, where he hopes the right lady will find him soon.

Carl Jahrstorfer (72) compared his journey to the movie *Cast Away*, where Tom Hanks plays the lone survivor of a plane crash, marooned on a tiny island in the Pacific. He says he felt lost at sea and in survival mode, sometimes talking to himself, dealing with disappointments, but always having faith. Carl recently relocated from Connecticut to North Carolina so he could be closer to his family. He continues to look for Mrs. Right.

Pastor Bob Page (71) remarried and continues to serve as an Associate Pastor at a church located in The Villages, Florida.

Robert Schlieper (64) plays a lot of golf, travels some, and remains an active member of the Widowers Support Network.

Widower Keith Meriam (59) feels grateful he had time to prepare for his wife Suzy's passing, as it gave them time to make preparations together. Keith says: "Grieve as long as you NEED to, and don't let anyone tell you how to do it. Then re-join the world and live your life as you know she would want you to." Keith married his new wife, Andrea, in 2001. They continue to live in Hawaii.

Tony Cabuno (50) tells us how it took a while for him to get back on his feet. "I realized the boys had lost a mother and they couldn't afford to lose their father as well." It was then that Tony decided that it was best for his family if they would attempt to move on with their everyday life, not dwelling on the past but rather looking toward the future. A few years later, Tony met his wife, Brittany. "Our life went from tragedy to fairytale," said Tony. "Today, my life could not be better."

When asked if he feels he has moved forward with his life, John Heffernan (59) says: "We are always moving forward, in my view. I don't necessarily see moving forward as requiring another female relationship; I am alone but not lonely. I stay very busy with friends, family, work, hobbies, and volunteering. I continue to feel like the luckiest guy in the world. I had over 30 years with the right partner. Most people never get that. I am grateful."

There you have it, *The Widower's Journey*, the culmination of my efforts over the past nine years to comfort and assist widowers. To the widowers who have just finished reading this book, I'll leave you with my favorite thought: Now is the time for you to celebrate your beloved wife's life by living yours.

APPENDIX I

Your Finances

A s if losing your wife weren't crisis enough, you may face a financial crisis because of her death. At the least, your finances may be in disarray and need an overhaul. Long months of caregiving means many men leave work, and that puts them in a financial hole. And the loss of her income after her death may put making payments on assets such as homes and cars in jeopardy. You may be responsible for a mountain of medical bills, and childcare expenses may mount if your kids are young and need extra attention.

So this appendix gives advice on managing your finances after your wife dies. I'll talk about first steps; how to collect money owed to you; how to protect your home; how to manage a life insurance payout; and special financial pitfalls a widower may face. When writing this appendix, I gratefully received advice from subject matter experts and financial planners Mark Colgan of Honeoye Falls, NY., and Jennifer Ferguson of Lake Mary, FL.

First, let me list some steps you need to take, roughly in chronological order:

1. **Order a minimum of 15 certified copies of the death certificate.** The funeral home can usually provide them.

2. **Empty your safe deposit box.** When you go to the bank to do so, there is no need to say that your wife is deceased. If you do mention that, it may require the bank to freeze the box, preventing you from entering it until a state official can be present.

3. **Contact each financial institution where your late wife banked.** Depending on the state in which you reside, and the title of the accounts held, you may then be required to obtain a release before funds can be withdrawn from those accounts. A bank officer can explain the procedure for obtaining a release. You will need to take a copy of the death certificate (a certified copy is preferred).

4. **Apply to receive death benefits.** Write formal letters notifying companies and organizations that your wife is deceased. Such organizations may include the Social Security Administration, the Veterans Administration, the deceased's employer or former employer, union, civil service, professional and trade associations, fraternity/sorority, alumni association, and even automobile club where she may have held an insurance policy. You may also qualify for burial allowances. The VA provides a marker for the grave, an American flag for the casket and, in some cases, a plot at a National Cemetery for both you and your deceased wife's burial. Contact your local U.S. National Cemetery for details. You can find a list of them at www.cem.va.gov/cems/listcem.asp.

5. **Collect on larger life insurance policies.** If your wife owned a life insurance policy, either you will receive the funds or—in the case of some insurance companies—you may be offered an opportunity to deposit the policy's proceeds into an interest-bearing account with the insurer. These accounts usually pay a market interest rate but are not likely to offer FDIC insurance. You also have the option to deposit the funds into a bank account as a temporary home until you

have time to determine how you would like to manage the money. My advice: Move the proceeds from the life insurance company. More on this later.

6. **Secure important papers and documents.** Certain documentation is needed to claim death benefits. Among the documents you will need to secure include but are not limited to: deeds; car titles; car registrations; insurance documents; vendor service contracts; wills; trusts; savings accounts; checking accounts; certificates of deposit; annuities; mutual funds; stocks; monthly and annual statements for brokerage accounts and bank accounts; and insurance policies for car, home, and any other real estate. Also, if your late wife had an accountant, check with them for business arrangements that you may not be aware of, as well as for tax records. Keep documents including life insurance policies and certificates, even if premiums haven't been paid for years. The policy may still be in force or have a cash value. Also, canceled checks and receipts may be needed to prove payment or ownership.

7. **If your deceased spouse had a retirement account (401(k), IRA, Roth IRA, etc.), find the paperwork and alert the company where the account is held (mutual fund, insurance company, bank, brokerage, etc.) of your wife's death.** But avoid cashing in such accounts without first consulting your tax advisor or fully understanding the consequences—the wrong decision may make you incur unnecessary taxes and penalties. In some cases, you can take out a loan against such accounts to help you pay bills in the short term.

8. **Notify all creditors to whom your spouse owed money, including installment loans, credit cards, mortgages, student loans, and service contracts.** Ask if any outstanding loans are insured, or if any life insurance benefits are due. Some loans may become fully paid in the event of a customer's

death, and some may not need to be paid, so don't be hasty to settle debts until you know all the terms. If medical bills are due, a hospital may hold the bills for 60 to 90 days.

9. **If a trust was established by your deceased spouse, discuss the terms of the trust with the trust officer.**
10. **Change the legal title of any joint property and other important documents (deeds, car titles, etc.) to your name alone, but check with your tax advisor before doing so.**
11. **If your children are attending college, contact their school's financial aid office.** When a parent dies, college students are often eligible for increased financial aid, loans, or grants.

Social Security

Especially when it comes to couples, Social Security benefits can be complicated. Contributing widower Steve Marquardt secured some financial assistance from the Social Security Administration, but only after enduring three appeals and then standing in front of a five-person board and fighting to receive something his wife had worked for and rightfully earned. Widowers facing similar challenges should contact an attorney who specializes in such matters.

After nearly four decades in the financial service industry, you would think I would know something about personal finances. While I picked up a tip or two along the way, the truth was, I was out of touch with Social Security. After all, I was only 57 when Michelle passed away. It wasn't until three years later, in 2010, that my sister called me and suggested I look into Social Security survivor benefits. She was right. At the age of 60, a widower is eligible for survivor benefits. And in my case, it was not an insignificant amount based on Michelle's contributions to Social Security over the years. My eligibility will remain in place until I finally decide to begin collecting on my own Social Security account once I reach the minimum eligibility age of 62, at which time the survivor benefits would stop.

While the Social Security Administration endeavors to do a good job, they are no different than most companies: It is staffed with some great representatives and some who are still learning the rules. Articles have been written on how some Social Security reps don't understand their own system.

There are several online tools that can assist widowers in making informed decisions when it comes to Social Security benefits. Among the ones I have come across is *Maximize My Social Security* (www.MaximizeMySocialSecurity.com). This highly rated website is a powerful yet simple-to-use financial tool.

However, this is no substitute for receiving advice from a financial planner or lawyer who is an expert in the best strategies for collecting Social Security benefits.

Your Home

The rate of foreclosures among widowed people is rising. There are several different factors contributing to this problem, not least of which is the rising level of consumer debt held by those paying mortgages, as well as the lack of a nest egg for handling unanticipated expenses. And of course, the loss of a second income can be a devastating blow to holding on to a home.

How did things get like this? Years ago, one wage earner was able to cover the financial needs of an average family. As time went on, families wanted larger homes, two cars in the driveway, etc., and that usually meant depending on the other spouse's income to help pay the bills.

Refinancing the mortgage to a monthly payment that the widower alone can afford can sometimes work. That means stretching out the length of the mortgage, but it also means keeping the home and avoiding the disruption of having to move after the loss of the spouse.

And as I detailed back in Chapter 1, be sure to apply for a home equity line of credit so that you'll be able to use the equity in your home for a loan in emergencies. The best time to do this is when the spouse is still alive and has an income.

Also, if you're 62 years old or older and own your house outright, or you have a low balance on your mortgage, another way to tap your home's equity is through a reverse mortgage. Under the provisions of a reverse mortgage, the borrower preserves the right to remain in the mortgaged home, and a portion of the home's equity is paid to the borrower each month, or you can receive it as a lump sum. Be sure to explore other options before committing to a reverse mortgage, because fees and interest rates can be high, your heirs may not get the house, and if you move you have to repay the loan. There are many strings attached. You've probably seen ads for them on TV. Contributing widower and financial expert Mark Colgan says, "Reverse mortgages are controversial products that only make sense in certain cases."

If paying a mortgage or paying for home maintenance is burdensome, downsizing may be an option. You may be able to buy a smaller home or a condo outright and not have to pay a mortgage at all.

Life Insurance

Let me take a moment to talk about life insurance and make a recommendation. When life insurance proceeds are paid out to a beneficiary, the insurance company's representative will often try to sell you an annuity or some other financial product, paid for by the proceeds of the insurance policy. They may even try to persuade you to keep your money with the company until you make a decision. Regardless, just get the settlement money and tuck it away in your bank or with your mutual fund company. Here's why: You may not need an insurance product at that point in your life. And if you do need an annuity (a contract in which you turn over a lump sum and get payments for life), you need to shop for the best annuity from among many insurance companies.

When awarding death benefits, many insurance companies use a sales tactic that requires you to meet with them at their office. They want to have you on their turf when they attempt to convince you to convert the life insurance proceeds to one of their products. They may even tell you "it is required" that you come to the insurance office to sign some papers. This is nonsense.

In my case, I was told I needed to come to the insurance office if I wanted to pick up the check. But having been in the financial services business for years, I knew better. Besides, my wife had recently died, I was recovering from kidney stone surgery, I had no interest in being sold anything, and I didn't want to make the trip. I called the agent back and told them to mail me the proceeds of Michelle's life insurance policy, or I was going to contact their compliance department and inform them of how I was treated. The check arrived by overnight mail. Not only was the agent wrong in saying I had to meet at his office but, in my view, he was also preying on a new widower.

Finding a Financial Planner

You may have never used a financial planner but find that you need one to help you sort out Social Security, mortgage, and other issues after your wife dies. Often widowers will need to buy new insurance policies and make arrangements for the care of their children under their new circumstances.

Books have been written about finding a planner, and I won't try to write a condensed one here. My general advice is to first find a true financial planner. Not a stock broker who has taken some classes and has a flimsy designation. Not an insurance agent with the same weak qualifications. For me, I prefer Certified Financial Planners (CFPs). I especially like the CFPs whose business is to provide advice on a fee-only basis, as it prevents conflicts of interest—they don't make a commission from selling me what they recommend that I purchase, so they're not tempted to sell me something that yields them a higher commission. They also won't churn my account with excessive transactions that also make them money. If you want to find a fee-only planner, the National Association of Personal Financial Advisors (www.napfa.org) can help you do so in your area.

When searching for a financial advisor, Colgan recommends that widowers look for the Five Cs:

- **Character:** Is the provider (or their firm) free of complaints or concerns filed by clients or regulators.
- **Commission:** What fees/commissions, etc. will you be expected to pay annually.
- **Client:** How many clients does the provider service? You want to be sure the provider has time to serve your needs.
- **Credentials:** What credentials does the provider possess?
- **Commitment:** Ask the provider to explain in detail why you should believe they're committed to servicing your needs.

As you can imagine, the fee schedules of financial advisors are all over the map, so you need to evaluate their costs against the value of their service. Typically, planners charge a one-time flat fee of $500 to $5,000 for the creation of a comprehensive financial plan. And you can expect an annual fee to keep the plan up to date.

Also, Colgan recommends that widowers consider using the online service offered by Everplans.com, a comprehensive end-of-life planning tool, complete with recommendations, resources, and checklists. After the user answers a few simple questions about himself, Everplans will create a customized set of planning "to-dos" and help you build an end-of-life plan that's custom-tailored to your situation. To learn more, see www.everplans.com.

After you have your financial plan in place and you understand what needs implementation, ask around for referrals to licensed insurance agents, investment sales representatives, attorneys or accountants. While I recommend fee-only planners when developing a plan, you'll still need help executing the plan you have just purchased. That's is where these folks come into play.

Look for professional designations such as CLU (Chartered Life Underwriter), ChFC (Chartered Financial Consultant), CASL (Chartered Advisor for Senior Living), RICP (Retirement Income Certified Professional), LUTCF (Life Underwriter Training Council Fellow). Check with your State insurance department and FINRA (Financial Industry Regulatory Authority) for background and experience information of the financial brokers, advisors, and firms you are considering using. Be sure to ask if there have been any "reportable events" related to those you are considering doing business with, as such reports may cause you to look elsewhere for services. Take your time and meet with at least two professionals from different firms. Get everything in writing. Whatever you do, don't be that guy who works everything up and files the information away in a drawer somewhere, never implementing the plan designed to protect their financial interests.

APPENDIX II

Your Legal Affairs

t amazes me how so many men fail to have the appropriate legal papers in place before a family crisis occurs. Just read what contributing widower Tony Cabuno shared with us after he and his wife, Dawn, failed to arrange for living wills or a last will and testament. "It made things difficult," said Tony. "I lost my home, and my credit is still screwed up, so I am in the process of going bankrupt. Then I had to sell my business, a bar, so I could take care of the kids." Proper estate planning may not have eliminated all of the challenges Tony faced during Dawn's illness or following her death, but it could have helped.

So in this appendix, we'll review how to select an attorney, what documents you'll need, and some legal strategies. This is just a general overview, and of course thick books have been written on just this subject. I strongly suggest you hire an attorney to help you with these affairs. To give you an idea of what you'll need to do we invited attorneys Diedre Wachbrit-Braverman of Boulder, Colorado and Sofia Guzman of North Lauderdale, Florida to comment.

I know that some widowers may want to handle drafting and then filing certain legal documents on their own in hopes of lessening their legal expenses. You can buy a variety of legal templates for documents such as wills, living wills, powers of attorney, etc. on various websites, such as Legalzoom.com. Legal forms are also available at stationery stores such as Staples and Office Depot. Those who chose this avenue will enjoy lower fees, but it may be penny wise and pound foolish. As a 38-year veteran of the financial services industry, I don't recommend it.

If you insist on going this route, you may want to have the completed documents reviewed by an attorney who is experienced in estate planning. Then arrange for the attorney to check your documents following any life-changing events such as the death of one of your heirs, or changes in your marital, financial, or career status.

Finding an Attorney

If you choose to use an attorney you'll want one who specializes in estate planning, trust, and probate law. Don't pick a lawyer who is a jack of all trades. Attorney Diedre Wachbrit-Braverman, an expert in all the specialties above, describes such attorneys as practicing "threshold law," meaning they say they can handle whatever steps over the threshold of their office door. "Their fee structure may be attractive and their results predictable—predictably bad."

You can contact your local bar association for referrals. When you do, I suggest you tell them, "My wife has died. I need to file a probate in our county. Which of your members has the most experience and the best record of success in estate planning, trust, and probate cases? Could you give me a few names?"

Braverman recommends interviewing more than one attorney and vetting attorneys with the Better Business Bureau to see if they have clean records. Also visit Avvo.com, an attorney-rating service, to look for attorneys in your vicinity with the best score out of 10. Avvo.com is an amalgamation of client reviews and colleague reviews. Braverman recommends an attorney who scores 8.5 or better.

Your first consultation with any attorney should be free, and during this meeting, you need to nail down fees. The most affordable attorney may not be your best choice; likewise, the priciest isn't necessarily the best. Braverman recommends asking for referrals from satisfied clients who had similar needs as you.

Legal and Estate Planning

With your wife gone, your legal situation regarding your will, who will take care of your children in the event of your death, and who will make medical decisions on your behalf may change dramatically. So you will need to change the necessary documents to adjust to your new situation.

Beyond updating your will, you need to consider the following documents: a HIPAA release, a durable power of attorney, and advance medical directives such as a healthcare power of attorney or a living will. Depending on your situation, your interests may also be served by establishing an estate plan that may include a trust (there are different types) along with a pour-over will. Not every widower is in need of completing each of the documents.

Attorney Guzman explains how a HIPAA release lets a designated person or entity have access to your medical records and enables them to consult with your doctors about your care.

A durable power of attorney lets you appoint a representative to handle specific legal and financial responsibilities. Attorney Braverman tells us that a durable power of attorney enables a widower's designee to make financial transactions on behalf of the widower should he become debilitated or otherwise too ill to handle such matters.

By having an advance medical directive in place, such as a living will, the grantor can instruct his medical care providers how he wishes to be treated when he is no longer able to articulate his wishes. Guzman says that, for example, a living will instructs "whether you do or do not want interventions such as cardiac resuscitation, artificial feeding and hydration, and mechanical ventilation."

With most types of living wills, you do not appoint a person to make healthcare decisions on your behalf. Because a living will cannot cover every health care situation that may arise, you should also have a healthcare power of attorney. A healthcare power of attorney is a document in which you appoint a person to be your agent (aka, proxy) to make all healthcare decisions on your behalf, should you become unable to do so. Your agent makes decisions according to your wishes, and if your wishes are unknown, your agent will decide based on what he or she thinks you would want. This, instead of having to accept the default policies of the hospital you are in, or even the best guess of your physician. Braverman says the healthcare power of attorney would not only name the person who will speak on your behalf, but it would also name one or more backups that you authorize to make medical decisions for you.

Guzman advises, "Having both a living will and a healthcare power of attorney provides the best protection for a person's treatment wishes."

Trusts and Pour-Over Wills

A trust is a legal layer that surrounds one's assets, like a bubble that allows you, or others you authorize, to have complete control over those assets, says Braverman. "A trust can be very helpful if you are concerned that your heirs may foolishly spend all they inherit." This concern frequently surfaces when the grantor of the trust has young children or grandchildren. You may wish to direct part of your estate to a favorite charity or not-for-profit, or you may have other special concerns, such as a need to prevent relatives you have had previous disagreements with from inheriting your estate or benefiting in any way from of your assets.

The most common type of trust used by widowers is a revocable living trust. Such a document allows the widower to still maintain control of his assets. Conversely, assets placed into a living trust are controlled by the trustee. Further, a revocable living trust enables the signor to avoid probate—a process which may alter how their estate is to be distributed. Probate can also be expensive.

Attorney Sofia Guzman explains how some widowers who create a revocable living trust to avoid probate may also want to establish a pour-over will. "A pour-over will simply states that any assets that have not been put into a person's revocable living trust at the time of the person's death, should be transferred to, or poured into the trust and distributed to the beneficiaries of the trust," she says.

If you do decide to establish a trust, you will need to appoint one or more trustees who will act on your behalf following your death. A trustee can be a friend or family member, your attorney, your accountant, or a colleague, for example. That being said, your trustee could also be a company that administers trusts or a trust company, many of which (but not all) are owned and operated by banks. A trust company can be a small regional firm or law office, or it could be a large national bank.

Once you chose your trustee, it is important that you discuss with them the details of your estate prior to your death. You also will want to negotiate what level of compensation he or she will receive for agreeing to serve. Braverman tells us, "You want to appoint someone with reliable judgment." It's also critical that your chosen trustee is financially sound. You don't want to place your trust in a person who might become tempted to misappropriate funds.

Protecting Children

Widowers with children who have yet to remarry are likely to leave their estate to their children. If the children are not of legal age, the widower may need to appoint a trustee (an individual or a trust company) to handle his affairs until such time as his intended children are of the age of majority, usually 21.

In some cases the widower may want to establish a trust to insure his wishes are honored and his children are provided for. Example: If all of a widower's estate is made available to a 21-year-old child, the child may spend it on cars or vacations when their father wanted them to save it for college tuition and expenses. In this case, the trust could disburse funds as needed to meet college expenses.

It is also important that widowers with surviving children make legal provisions for their children before establishing any relationship with a new woman, as doing otherwise may someday cause the disinheritance of a widower's children should the widower decide to remarry.

A widower with surviving children will need to appoint a guardian (and perhaps a backup guardian or two) for his children on the chance that he may die before his children reach the age of majority or adulthood. Should a widower die without having the appropriate legal documents in place, Child and Family Services or another state agency will likely take custody of any surviving children until an appropriate home is found for them, preferably with a member of the children's family. Again, this is a matter to be addressed by the widower's attorney.

One of the immediate needs for widowers is providing protection for the children's inheritances. The most obvious risk to the inheritance earmarked for surviving children is the remarriage of the children's father. While a widower may feel he is comfortable with his new love, and that she would not intentionally violate his wishes should he die, he needs to legally lock in his wishes.

A responsible widowed father who seeks to remarry should have a prenuptial agreement drafted. If she loves you, she'll understand your feelings and be more than happy to sign it for you. Besides, a prenuptial agreement can also protect your new love while providing some considerations or provisions intended to give her peace of mind and security.

Once you and your attorney have completed and executed the documents that will address your needs, be sure to have copies provided to those who should have access to them. It is also recommended that all widowers subscribe to the services of a registrar such as DocuBank.com or Legal Directive (LegalDirective.com). This will make your critical papers accessible when an emergency strikes, regardless of your location.

Braverman suggests that a widower should, at a minimum, do the following:

- Place his assets, if they exceed $300,000, into a revocable living trust before any relationship gets serious. This would include any death benefits from life insurance policies and retirement plans.
- If the widower plans to remarry, he should get a prenuptial agreement to protect his assets and make provisions for division of assets and spousal support should the marriage end in divorce.
- When a widower remarries, he needs to be careful not to let his new wife make a payment on his mortgage, his business, his investments, a car, or any asset of his. That's called commingling, and a single payment by her on your house can result in her inheriting the whole thing.
- A widower should not pay for any of his new wife's debts, as a court may rule that by doing so, he assumed the debt. If he wants to help her, he should give her a check with "gift" in the subject line and let her pay her bills.

APPENDIX III

Support From Pets

When considering what actions widowed men can take in hopes of accelerating their healing, they may only have to reach down to the pet seated beside them. I witnessed the power of pets often during Michelle's illness, especially during the final hours of her life when her son Jacques carried each of Michelle's three golden retrievers, one at a time, from his car up to her hospital room. The nursing staff placed a gurney beside Michelle's bed so her beloved Charlotte, Spencer, and Carolina could lie beside her one last time.

In this appendix, I'll discuss the positive benefit of pets, and also direct you to resources for pets that are specially trained to provide support and assistance.

My first exposure to the phenomenon of pet therapy was back in the 1990s when my bank duties included leading KeyBank of New York's annual Neighbors Make a Difference Day. On this day, the bank would close at noon to free up employees to go into the neighborhoods they served and perform community services. One time, bank volunteers took a group of dogs from the local animal shelter to a nearby nursing home. Some dogs were even invited by the seniors to jump up onto their beds. I still remember the looks of joy and comfort on the faces of the seniors when petting and playing with the dogs. Neither the home's residents nor the dogs wanted the visit to end.

According to the Mayo Clinic, "animal-assisted therapy (AAT) can significantly reduce pain, anxiety, depression and fatigue in people with a range of health problems including those suffering from post-traumatic stress disorder." AAT is the use of trained animals to assist patients in achieving established health objectives and is the first of two therapies grouped under the heading of Pet Therapy. The second is animal-assisted activities, which has a more general purpose, such as what the seniors experienced when the KeyBank volunteers visited them with the dogs."

The Paws for People website (www.pawsforpeople.org) adds: "It's well-known (and scientifically proven) that interaction with a gentle, friendly pet has significant benefits including releasing endorphins that have a calming effect and can diminish overall physical pain. The act of petting produces an automatic relaxation response, reducing the amount of medication some folks need, lifts spirits and lessens depression, encourages communication, lowers anxiety, reduces loneliness" and more.

Widower Mark R. Colgan had this to say about his two Labrador retrievers, Murray and Tucker: "The evening Joanne died my two Labradors proved to be more than companions, they were family members that were grieving the loss of Joanne. As I sat downstairs, reflecting on the day's shocking events, I heard an unusual cry coming from the bedroom. The bedroom that Joanne had died in earlier in the day. As I peered around the corner of the bedroom door, I saw how the cry was coming from one of our dogs, Murray. He lied on the bed in the spot Joanne had died and was crying in a way that I have never heard a dog cry before. He was mourning."

But it's not only dogs that provide us support and solace. Some widowers are more the cat-lover type, and similar benefits have been attributed to cats and other pets.

Professor Carr notes that pets serve another important purpose: they give widowers a schedule and routine. For many widowers, especially those who are retired, days can feel long and empty. Some widowers struggle to get out of bed. However, a dog eager for a walk or a cat meowing for her morning kibble force us to get out of bed, face the day, and set up routines that can be a healthy and important source of structure.

Therapy Dogs Versus Service Dogs

Sometimes there is confusion about which animals qualify as therapy dogs and which qualify as service dogs. They are not the same, though a dog may serve in both capacities. While a therapy dog brings comfort to those in need of companionship, service dogs have been "individually trained to do work or perform tasks for the benefit of a person with a disability," according to the Americans with Disabilities Act. These people would include those with either a mental or physical condition "which substantially limits a major life activity."

If you have disabilities and are hoping to acquire a dog that can perform tasks for you, then you need to apply for a service dog. Acquiring a service dog is a bit more complicated and expensive than getting a therapy dog. Don't let that dissuade you from considering a service dog, if that is what you actually need. If you are a physically challenged widower, a service dog can fill the role of both performing tasks you are unable or challenged to perform on your own and serving as the emotional therapy pet you may need.

Across America, there are many animal shelters, SPCAs, and civic, service, and charitable organizations that have programs that can assist in the acquisition of a proper animal, and some even contribute to the cost of doing so. You can call your local agencies and learn what is available, or check a master list provided by the

American Kennel Club. That list is available at www.akc.org/events/ title-recognition-program/therapy/organizations.

Here are some additional resources:

ESA Doctors (www.esadoctors.com). This website provides information about emotional support animals (ESAs) and how to secure one. Sign up for news, discounts, and activities.

Paws for People (www.pawsforpeople.org). A non-profit whose mission is to "provide elders, children, and folks with disabilities individualized, therapeutic visits with a gentle, affectionate pet."

Pet Partners (www.petpartners.org). "Pet Partners teams interact with a wide variety of clients including veterans with PTSD, seniors living with Alzheimer's, students with literacy challenges, patients in recovery, people with intellectual disabilities and those approaching end of life."

About the Author

Herb Knoll

Herb Knoll lost his wife, Michelle, to pancreatic cancer on March 7, 2008. Knoll is a retired bank executive, marketer, and professional speaker turned widower advocate. He founded the Michelle's Angels Foundation, Inc., a not-for-profit organization with a mission to "provide love, hope, compassion, and comforting music to those who quietly suffer" (MichellesAngel.com). Knoll also founded the Widowers Support Network in 2014 (WidowersSupportNetwork.com), so he could better serve, comfort, and assist widowers.

Knoll has previously served as a weekly columnist for the *Rochester Democrat & Chronicle*, a contributing writer for *Sales & Marketing Management* and *Marketing Times* magazines, and as an on-air talent for television commercials. As the former director of public and media relations for KeyBank (NY) and later as president of Marketplace Bank (FL), Knoll frequently appeared as his bank's spokesperson on radio and television. PBS affiliate WNED produced and aired the three-part series *Today's Executive*, featuring Herb's business insights, which were featured in his 1985 book, *The Total Executive*.

An inductee of the Buffalo/Niagara Sales & Marketing Executive's Hall of Fame, Knoll went on to serve as the Executive Director of the 10,000+ member Sales & Marketing Executives International and was a charter member of the board of directors for Nap Ford Community School in Orlando.

A former U.S. Army Reserve Drill Sergeant (E-7), Knoll is a proud member of the Knights of Columbus. Knoll lives in Lake Mary, Florida, with his wife, Maria.

About Deborah Carr, PhD

Having obtained her undergraduate degree from Connecticut College and her Ph.D. from the University of Wisconsin–Madison, Dr. Carr currently serves as Professor of Sociology and Acting Director of the Institute for Health, Health Care Policy & Aging Research at Rutgers University. She has previously held positions at the University of Michigan–Ann Arbor and the University of Wisconsin–Madison. Dr. Carr is an internationally known expert on widowhood and bereavement, is the editor of *Spousal Bereavement in Later Life* (Springer, 2006), and the author of many journal articles and book chapters, many of which focus on the psychological adjustment to widowhood and end-of-life issues. Her articles and chapters can be found at rci.rutgers.edu/~carrds.

Dr. Carr has authored several other books, including *Worried Sick: How Stress Hurts Us and How to Bounce Back* (Rutgers University Press, 2014). She is editor-in-chief of *Journal of Gerontology: Social Sciences* and sits on the editorial board of other academic journals. Dr. Carr is a former chair of the Section on Aging and the Life Course of the American Sociological Association and is a Fellow at the Gerontological Society of America and a member of the honorific Sociological Research Association.

About Robert L. Frick

A career financial and business journalist, Robert L. Frick has co-authored three books on personal finance and has a B.A. in Journalism and an M.B.A., both from the Pennsylvania State University. He has worked as a business reporter, including for *USA Today*, and a business editor for the *Democrat & Chronicle* in Rochester, New York. For 15 years he was a writer and senior editor for *Kiplinger's Personal Finance* magazine, where he developed an expertise in and wrote extensively about behavioral finance and investor psychology. He worked for two years for the Allianz Center for Behavioral Science and was the editorial director of a financial publishing firm in Northern Virginia.

Books of Interest

Adjusting to Your New Life

Getting Organized: Revised and Updated by Stephanie Winston (Warner Books, 2006). A handy guide that has been helping people manage their daily lives since 1978 is revised and updated to apply the principles of organization to today's lifestyles.

The Grief Recovery Handbook by John W. James & Russell Friedman (HarperCollins, 2009). 20th Anniversary Expanded Edition: The Action Program for Moving Beyond Death, Divorce, and Other Losses including Health, Career, and Faith.

Essential Survival Guide to Living on Your Own by Sharon B. Siepel (Howard Books, 2007). Provides you with how-to and hands-on instruction to make life less of a chore and more of an adventure.

How to Survive the Loss of a Love by Melba Clogrover, Ph.D., Harold Bloomfield M.D. & Peter McWilliams (1993). Discusses the variety of reactions that people experience because of the loss of a love and provides numerous recommendation for coping with pain and achieving comfort.

Making Loss Matter by Rabbi David Wolke (2000). During moments of loss, "we must make a choice: Will we allow the difficulties we face to become forces of destruction in our lives, or will we find a way to begin learning from loss, transforming our suffering into a source of strength?"

Rays of Hope in Times of Loss by Susan Zimmerman (Expert Publishing, Inc., 2005). *Rays of Hope In Times of Loss* offers soothing guidance to help you discover the answer to many questions.

The Widower's Toolbox by Gerald Schaefer (New Horizon Press, 2010). *The Widower's Toolbox* offers men who have lost their partners a guide to help identify and resolve the issues overwhelming them and to repairing their lives and moving forward.

Two Kisses for Maddy by Matthew Logelin (2012). A story of love and recovery following the death of a man's wife, just twenty-seven hours after she gave birth to their beautiful daughter Madeline.

Caregiving

Caregiving without Regrets by Dr. Vicki Rackner *(Medical Bridges, 2009)*. For the newfound role as a caregiver, this book provides tips and action steps to help you serve.

Don't Take My Grief Away from Me by Doug Manning and Glenda Stansbury (In-Sight Books, 2003). The authors take the reader through all the emotions and experiences that accompany the death of a loved one.

In Lieu of Flowers by Nancy Howard Cobb (Pantheon Books, 2000, 2001). The author meets death in the most vital of places—in the lives of everyday people—and in doing so has found a way to infuse this darkest subject with light.

Into the Cave: When Men Grieve by Dr. Ronald G. Petrie (2001). *When Men Grieve* is a book that identifies the differences between the way men and women grieve.

Living Through Mourning: Finding Comfort and Hope When a Loved One Has Died by Harriet Sarnoff Schiff (1987). The Author shares advice to help mourners find comfort amidst grief and hope when a loved one has passed.

To Live Until We Say Goodbye by Elisabeth Kubler-Ross (A Touchstone Book, 1992). The methods of Dr. Kubler-Ross, the world-renowned psychiatrist, and authority on death, are revealed in this exploration of her counseling work with terminal patients to help them come to an acceptance of death.

Dating/Relationships

Dating A Widower by Abel Keogh (Ben Lomond Press, 2011). Drawing on his own experience as a widower who's remarried, Abel Keogh gives you unique insight into the hearts and minds of widowers.

Second Wives, the Pitfalls and Rewards of Marrying Widowers and Divorced Men by Susan Shapiro Barash (2000). This compassionate and timely guide to remarriage mixes insights and advice from experts with interviews with more than 100-second wives.

Financial Matters

The Survivor Assistance Handbook by Mark Colgan, CFP (2002, 2003, 2007, 2009). An invaluable reference for anyone experiencing the loss of a spouse or partner. Effectively manage the mountain of paperwork that follows death and safeguards your financial future by making better and smarter decisions about the estate.

Grief

Beyond Anger: A Guide for Men: How to Free Yourself from the Grip of Anger and Get More Out of Life by Thomas Harbin (Marlowe & Company, 2000) *Beyond Anger* shows the angry—and miserable—man how to change his life and relationships for the better.

On Grief and Grieving by Elizabeth Kubler-Ross (Scribner, 2014). *On Grief and Grieving* combines practical wisdom, case studies, and the authors' own experiences and spiritual insight to explain how the process of grieving helps us live with loss.

Swallowed by a Snake: the Gift of the Masculine Side of Healing by Tom Golden (G. H. Publishing LLC, 1997, 2010). It's a book for men and women about the masculine side of healing from loss.

The Way Men Heal by Thomas Golden (G.H. Publishing, LLC, 2014). *The Way Men Heal* is a concise book that offers insight into the masculine side of healing.

When A Man Faces Grief /A Man You Know Is Grieving by James E. Miller (Willowgreen Publishing, 1998). Two books in one. One-half is for men who are grieving, with 12 helpful suggestions, each a chapter by itself. The other half is for those who want to understand and help men who are grieving, also in twelve short, helpful chapters.

When Bad Things Happen to Good People by Harold Kushner (Anchor Books, 2004). *When Bad Things Happen to Good People* is a classic that offers clear thinking and consolation in times of sorrow.

When Men Grieve by Elizabeth Living (Fairview Press, 1998). *When Men Grieve* explains the special ways that men grieve so those who love them can better understand what they're going through.

Widower: When Men Are Left Alone by Scott Campbell and Phyllis R. Silverman (1996). A journalist and a social worker explore the grief process as men experience it.

Journeys Lived

Men Bleed Too by Thomas Brown (iUniverse, Inc., 2005). A man recounts the pain he endures during his wife's illness and her eventual death.

Walk With Me by Patricia Jahrstorfer (Xulongpress, 2013). In an age when so many have been touched by cancer, *Walk with Me* shares personal insights into how faith and medicine can exist side by side. Carl Jahrstorfer, the author's husband, completed this book following Patricia's death and is one of the contributing widowers to *The Widower's Journey*.

Widow-Man—A Widower's Story and Journaling Book by Dr. Nyle Kardatzke (2014). Though widowed men have much in common with widows, their journey is uniquely male. The author shares his practical responses to many issues faced by widowed men, including grief, changed relationships, anger, forgiveness, cooking, housekeeping, holidays and weekends, steps toward healing, and more. Author Dr. Nyle Kardatzke is one of the contributing widowers to *The Widower's Journey*.

Surviving Children

Talking About Death: A Dialogue Between Parent and Child by Earl A. Grollman (Beacon Press, 2011). How do you explain the loss of a loved one to a child? This book is a compassionate guide for adults and children to read together, featuring a read-along story and answers to questions children ask about death.

When Parents Die by Edward Myers (Penguin Group, 1997). Topics range from psychological responses to a parent's death, such as shock, depression, and guilt, to practical consequences, such as dealing with estates and funerals.

Printed in Great Britain
by Amazon

44722237R00131